THE

MEDICAL LIBRARY ASSOCIATION

Consumer Health Reference Service Handbook

by **DONALD A. BARCLAY**
and **DEBORAH D. HALSTED**

NEAL-SCHUMAN PUBLISHERS, INC.
NEW YORK **LONDON**

Published by Neal-Schuman Publishers, Inc.
100 Varick Street
New York, NY 10013

The paper used in this publication meets minimum requirements of American National Standard for Information Sciences—Permanence of Paper for Printed Library Materials, ANSI Z39, 48–1992.

Printed and bound in the United States of America.

ISBN: 1–55570–418–2

Library of Congress Cataloging-in-Publication Data

Barclay, Donald A.
      The Medical Library Association consumer health reference service handbook /
Donald A. Barclay, Deborah D. Halsted.
            p.   cm.
         1. Health—Information services—Handbooks, manuals, etc. 2. Medicine—
Information services—Handbooks, manuals, etc. 3. Medicine, Popular—Handbooks,
manuals, etc. I. Title: Consumer health reference service handbook. II. Halsted,
Deborah. III. Medical Library Association. IV. Title.

RA776 .B234 2001
025.06'61—dc21

                                                                                    2001037051

Dedication

This book is dedicated to my husband, Robert T. Murray, and to my parents Albertine (Waggi) and Benjamin D. Halsted for their love and support.
—Deborah D. Halsted

I would like to dedicate this book to Darcie and Tess. Good health to you.
—Donald A. Barclay

Contents

List of Figures

Preface

The Medical Library Association Consumer Health Reference Service Handbook is designed as a practical guide for librarians facing the enormously challenging job of helping patrons find accurate and authoritative answers to health questions. Anyone who works a reference desk serving any segment of the general public can tell you that answering consumer-health questions[1] makes up a big part of the workload. Typically, from 5 to 10 percent of all questions at a public library reference desk involve consumer-health,[2] and finding answers to such questions is time consuming, often requiring 20 minutes or more per question.[3] But such numbers, while significant, do not tell the whole story of how challenging finding answers to consumer-health questions can be.

Conducting an effective reference interview with people with consumer-health questions demands special attention. Users are often unsure of what information they need. Perhaps they saw a television news segment or advertisement about a medication that might help their asthma, but they aren't sure what the medication is called. Maybe they need information about some biomedical mouthful of a disease that they can hardly pronounce, much less spell. The desire for privacy complicates these basic reference tasks and can make it difficult for a library patron to explicitly describe their consumer-health information needs. Who, after all, would feel comfortable going to a public place to ask a complete stranger for information on hemorrhoids, erectile dysfunction, hair lice, or any of a host of stigmatized diseases and conditions?

Even when those seeking information can clearly state their information need, finding answers to health questions can be quite stressful to the professional charged with the task. Directing someone to an inappropriate source of health information—or flat-out failing to find relevant information—can have consequences much more dire than routine reference referrals. Adding to the stress is the always-lurking concern about when, exactly, helping consumers

---

1. By "consumer health information," we mean any health-related information intended for the general public as opposed to information intended for health professionals. Of course the line between the two types of information is not always clear, and it is quite common for members of the general public to use information intended for health professionals to answer consumer health questions.
2. See pages 188–189 of Dewdney, Patricia, Joanne G. Marshall, and Muta Tiamiyu. "A Comparison of Legal and Health Information Serices in Public Libraries." *RQ.* 31(2): 185–196. Winter 1991.
3. See page 45 of Earl, Martha. "A Medical Library Reaches Out to Help the Public Answer Their Health Care Questions." *American Libraries.* 29(10): 44–46. November 1998.

find health-related information becomes practicing medicine without a license. How do you handle the prospect of a disgruntled patron wanting to sue you and your library because you provided bad health information? On top of all this, health-related questions can be emotionally wrenching. If helping a stressed-out undergraduate find information for a term paper (due tomorrow) is tough, helping a tearful mother find information about malignant brain tumors in children under the age of five is off the scale.

Audience

The Medical Library Association Consumer Health Reference Service Handbook is a primer on consumer-health librarianship designed for librarians and others who help the general public locate consumer-health information. The collateral audience for this book is clinicians, social workers, health-department employees, and others who work with members of the public who need, or could benefit from, access to consumer-health information.

Purpose

As the amount of available information on consumer health explodes so too does the need for one comprehensive guide to help the overworked professionals that assist the public who searches it. Librarians need to not only make sense of the content but also assist users to utilize it as intelligently, efficiently, and successfully as possible. *The Medical Library Association Consumer Health Reference Service Handbook* shows how to understand information and terminology, cull the best resources, and provide capable yet compassionate reference services. *The Handbook* then offers innovative ideas to customize consumer health for the needs of individual libraries. Each of these large subjects is organized concisely into this one easy-to-understand, essential guide. The information is organized to work independently — each chapter and each section can certainly be consulted separately — or read cover to cover. All of the parts together offer a logical, step by step, approach for hardworking professionals to understand consumer health information today and then suggest the best way to offer it to users.

Providing the public with consumer-health information is a tough job and *The Medical Library Association Consumer Health Reference Service Handbook* tries to help librarians become good at providing sound information and to feel comfortable doing it. It covers standard resources for answering health-related questions, discusses the art of the health-reference interview, and touches on such related matters as the legal implications of providing health information to consumers. Without giving short shrift to the many indispensable printed consumer-health information resources, it places a heavy emphasis on the use and evaluation of electronic health-information resources.

Another aim of *The Medical Library Association Consumer Health Reference Service Handbook* is to help librarians and others develop better consumer-health information services. Covering such topics as how to create an effective and useful consumer-health Web site; how to promote consumer-health information resources and services through outreach; and how to collaborate with health agencies and healthcare providers to improve access to consumer-health information. The CD-ROM component of this book includes a template for developing an effective consumer-health Web site and templates for designing in-house consumer-health information brochures.

The *Handbook* begins with Part 1, "Consumer Health Essentials for Librarians." The first chapter decodes medical terminology by clarifying the differences between types of health professionals, translates basic medical terminology, and illuminates common pharmaceutical names. Chapter 2, "Understanding Consumer Health Concerns," provides a concise explanation and essential background to the topics of the greatest interest to patrons. The list includes asthma, breast cancer, diabetes, high blood pressure, and dozens more of the top user concerns. In the third chapter it addresses the innovative and engaging areas of complementary and alternative medicine; exploring the hands-on therapies of acupuncture, chiropractic, osteopathy, massage therapy, and body work. Next the *Handbook* sheds light on some of the most popular mind-body therapies — relaxation techniques, meditation, hypnotherapy, biofeedback and spiritual healing. This chapter ends with an examination of herbal healing and lifestyle approaches, including homeopathy, herbs and botanicals, and dietary supplements.

Part 2 "Consumer Health Resources for Librarians," is designed as a complete basic resource and reference toolbox. It begins with the Internet, an area of primary interest to consumers. Chapter 4, "Recommended Consumer Health Web Sites," steers you through the often-complicated labyrinth of sites currently available on the Internet. After examining hundreds of sites, we culled over eighty of the best. We looked for expert content, useful links, and online services as well as considering features of the Web site itself: uniqueness, navigability, quantity, quality, and popularity. These reliable sites are presented alphabetically – everything from Achoo to Yahoo – and cover the great spectrum of important health concerns. As an added bonus on the CD-ROM, each of these recommended Web sites and cross-referenced lists are hyperlinked for easy access and possible downloadability.

As all experienced reference librarians know, the Internet, while certainly an essential element of health research, is only one part of the entire picture. The second part of *The Medical Library Association Consumer Health Reference Service Handbook* continues with Chapter 5, "Recommended Consumer Health Print Resources." Here we suggests ways to select the best books and publications and offer the specific titles that are particularly useful for a variety of health issues concerning users — including AIDS, Alzheimer's disease, heart disease, and liver disease. We also select the best publications on the interesting issues users seek information on. Our list includes women's and men's health, nutrition and exercise, fertility and sexuality, and reference among others. The last tools in this resource and reference section are offered in Chapter 6, "Recommended Consumer Health Resources About and For Children." In the first part we examine the best resources available about the health of children. In the second half we provide the key to the most useful health resources children themselves may want to explore.

Many librarians are exploring the innovative and exciting endeavor of creating customized services. Part 3, "Consumer Health Services for Librarians" will help as you enter or expand your services in this arena. Chapter 7 researches how to create these services. It investigates everything from collaboration between public and medical libraries, to malpractice and liability, to successful marketing. Chapter 8 discusses the best approaches to evaluating consumer health resources for your users. Chapter 9 shows how to create effective print consumer health publications for your users, focusing on how to write, lay out, and distribute your own print resources. In the last chapter, "Building Successful Consumer Health Web Sites for Your Users" the *Handbook* begins by exploring the basics of the customized site. It investigates ways to provide quality content while following standard design rules. It even includes a discussion of ways to draw attention to your site.

Providing patrons with practical consumer health information is a formidable task. It can also be one of the most rewarding reference encounters when accomplished with a sense of excitement, expertise, and expectation. We hope that *The Medical Library Association Consumer Health Reference Service Handbook* helps you locate the best resources and develop the finest skills to do the job well.

How to Use the CD-ROM

The CD-ROM includes two sections:

1. Recommended Consumer health Web Sites
2. The Hathaway Medical Center Library Consumer health Web site

Recommended Consumer Health Web Sites is a Web-ready HTML version of Chapter 4, "Recommended Consumer health Web Sites." Readers are welcome to cut and paste from this file in order to build their own lists of recommended Web sites.

The Hathaway Medical Center Library Consumer Health Web Site is a model consumer health Web site. Although the Hathaway Medical Center is fictional, this site can be used as a template to build your own customized site or give readers a very real idea of what kinds of information belong on a consumer health Web site and how such Web sites might be laid out.

The Hathaway Medical Center Library Web site consists of 18 Web pages, three .pdf files, and five images. Some of the pages have actual information on them, while others simply suggest how such a page might function without providing actual information. (The later type of page will have typesetter psuedo-Latin—"Lorem ipsum dolor sit..."—as filler text.) The starting point for this model Web site is its home page, which is title **index.html**.

A breakdown of the pages on the site follows:

about.html

Shows what can go on a typical "About" page. Experienced Web surfers know to look for the "About" page when they want information about the people behind the Web page or the organization the Web page represents.

diseases.html

A typical consumer health page that leads readers to reliable information about specific diseases and conditions. Such pages can consist of links to other Web sites or to locally produced information about disease and conditions of special interest to the local community or the organization which created the Web site.

faq.html

Commonly found on the Web, "frequently asked questions" pages provide answers to common questions. Experienced Web surfers know to look for the FAQ page when they need an answer to a basic question such as "Can non-doctors use your library?" or "How can I find medical information written in plain English?"

finding.html

This page provides library users with basic information on how to find consumer health information within the library itself.

hatahwaymc.html

This is the home page of the Hathaway Medical Center Library's parent institution. It falls into the category of "How Not to Do a Home Page."

hours.html

An example of an important—but often overlooked—page for any library Web site.

html.html and pdf.pdf

These are both "filler pages" designed to represent two versions of an imaginary user guide entitled "Guide to Finding Consumer Health Information in the Hathaway Medical Center Library." The page entitled **html.html** represents the version designed to be read on the Web, while the page entitled **pdf.pdf** represents the version designed to be printed.

html2.html and pdf2.pdf

These are both "filler pages" designed to represent two versions of an imaginary user guide entitled "Evaluating Consumer Health Information." The page entitled **html2.html** represents the version designed to be read on the Web, while the page entitled **pdf2.pdf** represents the version designed to be printed.

html3.html and pdf3.pdf

These are both "filler pages" designed to represent two versions of an imaginary user guide entitled "Lead-Based Paint: A Resource Guide for Residents of the Tri-County Area." The page entitled **html3.html** represents the version designed to be read on the Web, while the page entitled **pdf3.pdf** represents the version designed to be printed.

index.html

This is the home page for the Web site.

library.html

This page is entitled "Using the Hathaway Medical Center Library" and is intended to suggest what a Web page might contain to familiarize healthcare consumers with a health library.

local.html

This page suggests the kind of local information that might go on a consumer health Web site; a topic covered in some detail in the chapter on creating consumer health Web pages.

mission.html

This page would contain an institution's mission statement. Providing your mission statement is an effective way to tell Web visitors about your organization and its purpose.

policy.html

This page contains a sample disclaimer and privacy policy. A page of this type is a must for any Web site that provides health-related information.

pubs.html

A publications page such as this one is a good way to help users locate and obtain copies of any publications your institution provides via the Web.

sitemap.html

A good sitemap helps visitors see at a glance what is on a Web-site. Sitemaps are especially useful for visitors who, for whatever reason, cannot find what they are looking for by following the organizational scheme of a Website.

staff.html

This page, which is often a sub-page of the "About" page, is the place to list staff and departmental phone numbers, e-mail addresses, and physical addresses.

web.html

This page provides an example of a typical "Search the Web" page found on consumer health Web sites.

Introduction

What we today call "consumer health information" has long been a staple of the publishing industry. In centuries past, titles such as *Every Man His Own Doctor*[1] were nearly as common, and perhaps as frequently opened, as the family Bible. Over time, as printed matter got cheaper, literacy spread, and long lifetimes of good health became more common, consumer health books grew increasingly popular, a fact demonstrated today by bookstore shelves crowded with works on consumer health topics. At any full-service bookstore (whether brick-and-mortar or online) readers can find information on diet, exercise, medication, alternative medicine, and mental health; on how to cope with ailments ranging from the common cold to cystic fibrosis; on maintaining the health of every anatomical system from the skeleton to the thyroid; on helping the child grow up healthy and the adult stay young.

In Colonial America, a farmer might have purchased a book like *Every Man His Own Doctor* because trained medical help was too distant or expensive. Perhaps the farmer simply did not trust doctors, few of whom offered treatments any more sophisticated than what could have been provided by an experienced farmwife. Today, distance from trained healthcare professionals is rarely a problem (at least for those living in the industrialized world), but the cost of medical care remains a force that drives ordinary individuals to seek out relatively cheap healthcare information before—or instead of—seeking care from a professional. And, just as in the past, distrust of the medical establishment fuels the popularity of consumer health information, especially that which deals with alternative medicines and therapies.

Even when *distrust* is too strong a word to describe one's feelings about the healthcare establishment, more and more individuals are seeking out healthcare information so that they can become active participants in their healthcare decisions.

The rise of the Health Maintenance Organization (HMO) has also contributed to the current demand for consumer health information. The very nature of the HMO demands that patients who expect anything more than simple annual checkups become knowledgeable about their healthcare options. And because the HMO system often forces doctors to spend less time with patients, patients now turn to sources of consumer health information for answers to questions that, in the past, they might have asked their doctors.

---

1. Tennent, John. *Every Man his own Doctor: or, the Poor Planter's Physician.* The earliest extant copy (which is from the second edition) is dated 1734 and was printed in Williamsburg, Virginia. The book when through at least eight editions.

The Computer Transforms Consumer Health Reference

As popular as consumer health books (and magazine articles) are, the big news in consumer health information today is the Internet. Health-related information always ranks among the top types of information sought by Internet users:

- A 1998 survey of 1,000 Internet users found that 38 percent had searched the Internet for health-related information within the previous 12 months.[2]
- A Harris Poll published in March 2000 found that some 70 million people (nearly 75 percent of the online population) had used the Internet in the previous 12 months to find health-related information.[3]
- A survey of 100,000 Internet users published in April 2000 found that 3 percent shop online for health-related products.[4]

If a lot of people are using the Internet to search for health information, then it is not surprising that there is a lot of information out there for them to find. For example, **Yahoo!: Diseases and Conditions**[5] lists 7,298 Web pages devoted to everything from acne to Yunis-Varon Syndrome. The National Library of Medicine's **MEDLINE***plus*[6] provides extensive, carefully evaluated information on over 700 consumer health topics. Commercial healthcare giants like **drkoop.com**[7], **WebMD**[8], and **InteliHealth**[9] spend millions promoting their Web presences to potential visitors. A search of **Liszt, The Mailing List Directory**[10] retrieves 321 Internet mailing lists with the world "health" somewhere in their title. Entering such terms as "osteoporosis," "heart disease," or "diabetes" into any major Web search engine returns hundreds of thousands of hits on each term.

The Internet is a bountiful resource for health information, one with the potential to bring accurate, up-to-date health information to millions at little or no cost to the end user. There are, however, downsides to the Internet as a

2. Brown, Michael S. "Healthcare Information Seekers Aren't Typical Internet Users." *Medicine on the Net*. February 1998; 4(2): 17-18.
3. Wellner, Alison Stein. "Casting the Health .net." *American Demographics*. March 2000; 22(3): 46-49.
4. Zbar, Jeffery D. "Pharmacies Surge Online." *Advertising Age*. April 3, 2000; 71(14): S8-S10.
5. http://dir.yahoo.com/Health/Diseases_and_Conditions/
6. http://www.nlm.nih.gov/medlineplus/
7. http://drkoop.com/
8. http://webmd.com/
9. http://www.intelihealth.com/
10 .http://www.liszt.com/

source of health information. First of all, not everyone has Internet access or knows how to find information in an electronic environment. More significantly, there is a lot of potentially harmful health information on the Internet. An article published in *JAMA* in 1998 found that some of the health-related information on the Internet has the potential to harm the public by:

- causing individuals to seek inappropriate treatment or to delay seeking treatment
- making misleading claims for medical products
- spreading incorrect or inappropriate information through the medium of online support groups[11]

Whether the harmful health information on the Internet is there because of bad science, ignorance, zealotry, or greed, all of it has the potential to bring unnecessary pain or death to unsuspecting Internet users.

What all this adds up to for librarians, clinicians, medical social workers, and others who help put the public in touch with health information is more healthcare consumers looking for information, more places for them to find it, and more interested parties clamoring for the attention (and, sometimes, the money) of all those consumers. This begs the question: "What do we do about all this?"

New questions arise for professionals attempting to answer patrons questions about consumer health. How do we respond to following questions?

In a Web-crazed world where important new information resources seem to pop up every day, how do we familiarize ourselves with the most important, time-tested information resources in the field? How can we learn as much as we can about locating and evaluating consumer health information and find ways of teaching the members of the general public how to locate and evaluate such information for themselves? What are the best ways to cultivate our skills at conducting the consumer health reference interview while, at the same time, becoming comfortably aware of those legal and ethical boundaries we cannot cross when working with seekers of consumer health information? How do we develop complete consumer health information services through the creation of Web pages and printed guides as well as through partnerships with consumer health agencies and organizations?

The Medical Library Association Consumer Health Reference Service Handbook was written to confront these questions in your own library. It is intended to be a clear, concise, and concrete source of help in your own library or information center.

---

11. Robinson TN, Patrick K, Eng TR, Gustafson D. "An Evidence-Based Approach to Interactive Health Communication: A Challenge to Medicine in the Information Age. Science Panel on Interactive Communication And Health." *JAMA: The Journal of the American Medical Association.* October 14, 1998; 1280(14): 1264-9.

Acknowledgments

I would like to thank my father, Benjamin D. Halsted, for the hours he spent proofreading various drafts. Additionally, his advice as a health consumer was invaluable during the writing of the book.

—Deborah D. Halsted

I am grateful to my colleagues at the Houston Academy of Medicine-Texas Medical Center Library for giving their knowledge and friendship.

—Donald A. Barclay

PART I

Consumer Health
Essentials for Librarians

1
Decoding Medical Terminology

One of the most frustrating aspects of searching for information on any health topic is the terminology. From the different types of health professionals who assess your health data or treat your wounds, to the confusing words used to describe your condition, treatment, or cure, to the multiple names of pharmaceuticals and generic drugs, consumers and librarians alike may throw up their hands when confronted with this tower of babble. The purpose of this chapter is to help readers to decipher some of the "medspeak" that might be encountered when consumers seek health information.

Health Professionals

The term *doctor* is defined in *Dorland's Illustrated Medical Dictionary* as "a practitioner of the healing arts, one who has received a degree from a college of medicine, osteopathy, chiropractic, optometry, podiatry, pharmacology, dentistry, or veterinary medicine, licensed to practice by a state."[1] The same dictionary defines *physician* as "an authorized practitioner of medicine, as one graduated from a college of medicine or osteopathy and licensed by the appropriate board."[2] Simple enough. Unfortunately, the entire alphabet soup of medical terminology gets even more complicated when you address the issue of internship versus residency. An *intern* is "a graduate of a medical or dental school serving in a hospital preparatory to being licensed to practice medicine or dentistry,"[3] and generally refers to the first year of training after medical school. A *resident* is "a graduate and licensed physician receiving training in a specialty in a hospital."[4]

Most of the terms used in the *Dorland's* definition of doctor are recognizable, or easily defined with a medical dictionary. One term, *osteopathy*, is more confusing. Often, patients are not aware that their doctor is a Doctor of Osteopathy (DO) as opposed to a more recognizable Doctor of Medicine (MD) or allopathic physician. Allopathy is the type of medicine or system of therapeutics in which diseases are treated by creating a condition incompatible

---

1. *Dorland's Illustrated Medical Dictionary.* 29th ed. Philadelphia: W. B. Saunders, 2000. p. 539.
2. *Ibid.,* p. 1385.
3. *Ibid.,* p. 909.
4. *Ibid.,* p. 1558.

with the condition to be cured.[5] So what is a DO? The American Osteopathic Association explains that DOs are complete physicians, licensed by state and specialty boards to perform surgery and prescribe medication. Both DOs and MDs attend four-year undergraduate programs with an emphasis in science and four years of basic postgraduate medical education. Both types of physician complete a residency program, which takes between two and four years, and practice in fully accredited and licensed hospitals and medical centers. So what is the difference? Osteopathic schools emphasize training students to be primary care physicians in such areas as pediatrics, general practice obstetrics and gynecology, and internal medicine; in addition, DOs practice a "whole person" approach to medicine. Instead of treating specific symptoms or illnesses, they regard the patient's body as an integrated whole. Osteopathic physicians focus on preventive health care, especially by studying the musculoskeletal system. Many DOs fill a critical need for family doctors by practicing in small towns and rural areas.

Finally, many physicians are board certified, which means they have successfully completed an accredited training program and have passed a board examination in a particular specialty. Being board certified allows a physician to advertise himself or herself as a specialist in a particular field. To be eligible for board certification, residents need to successfully complete an accredited training program. Board-certified physicians are listed in the four-volume annual *Official ABMS Directory of Board Certified Medical Specialists.*[6]

Although there are many types of health professionals, one type that almost everyone encounters is nurses. Again, there are different types of nurses, including the two most common, licensed practical nurses (LPNs) and registered nurses (RNs). LPNs train for one year in state-approved programs, predominantly in vocational or technical schools. Their training includes both classroom study and supervised clinical practice (patient care). They are required to pass a licensing examination after completion of this program. LPNs provide basic bedside care, including taking vital signs (blood pressure, temperature, and respiration), prepare and give injections and enemas, collect samples from patients, and help patients with bathing, dressing, and personal hygiene. The majority of LPNs work in hospitals, with others working in nursing homes and doctors' offices.[7] RNs must graduate from a four-year nursing program and pass a national licensing examination to obtain a nursing license. RNs work to promote health, prevent disease, and help patients cope with illness. They are advocates and health educators for patients, families, and communities. When providing direct patient care they observe, as-

5. Ibid., *p. 51.*

6. *The Official ABMS Directory of Board Certified Medical Specialists.* Evanston, Ill.: American Board of Medical Specialties, Research and Education Foundation, 2000.

7. *Occupational Outlook Handbook.* Indianapolis: JIST Works, 2000. p. 227.

sess, and record symptoms, reactions, and progress; assist physicians during treatments and examinations; administer medications; and assist in convalescence and rehabilitation.[8]

Another type of health professional most people encounter is the pharmacist—the person who dispenses the drugs prescribed by physicians and other health professionals. Pharmacists, understanding the use, composition, and clinical effects of drugs, also advise physicians about medications and their use. Pharmacists, who may work in retail pharmacies, hospitals, or clinics, must have a license to practice pharmacy. To obtain a license, the pharmacist must graduate from an accredited college of pharmacy, serve an internship under a licensed pharmacist, and pass a state examination.[9]

To decode the often bewildering sets of initials that trail after the names of health professionals, consult:

Glossary of Health-Professional Titles
www.arthritis.org/alttherapies/default.asp#Glossary

Jablonski, Stanley. *Dictionary of Medical Acronyms & Abbreviations. 3d ed.* Philadelphia: Hanley & Belfus, 1998.

Davis, Neil M. *Medical Abbreviations: 14,000 Conveniences at the Expense of Communications and Safety.* 9th ed. Huntingdon Valley, Pa.: Neil Davis and Associates, 1999.

Basic Terminology

Besides discerning the difference between the various types of health professionals, probably the most intimidating aspect of doing consumer health research is the medical terminology itself. According to Fritz Spiegl:

> Doctors are obliged to learn a huge vocabulary. They need to have more words at their command than any philosopher, mathematician, engineer or astronomer. It is a daunting prospect for the medical student that apart from the manual and observational skills he must learn he is also required to be a polyglot linguist—for most of the essential words of his trade are foreign. The Doctor's professional vocabulary is constructed chiefly from Latin and Greek (or a mixture of the two).[10]

---

8. *Ibid.*, pp. 210–211.
9. *Ibid.*, pp. 203–204.
10. Spiegl, Fritz. *Sick Notes: An Alphabetical Browsing Book of Derivations, Abbreviations, Mnemonics and Slang for the Amusement and Edification of Medics, Nurses, Patients and Hypochondriacs.* New York: Parthenon, 1996. p. ix.

When a librarian, patient, or caregiver tries to do research on a medical condition, medical terminology must be understood at a certain level. Even though a wealth of consumer health information is available from books, databases, and Web sites, all of these sources use medical terminology to one extent or another. Additionally, many medical conditions require the researcher to access databases created for the health professionals, and the highly technical medical terminology one encounters is daunting.

Medical terms can generally be broken down into word parts, including roots, prefixes, suffixes, and linking or combining vowels. The root of a word is the part that contains the essential meaning of the word. It can also be thought of as the foundation of the term. For example, in the term *pericarditis*, the root word is *card*, which refers to the heart. The prefix *peri*, which adds to the root word, means "surrounding." The suffix *–itis* is a little more difficult, but means "inflammation." Almost all medical terms have a suffix. A common suffix is *–ology* or "the study of." Therefore, by breaking down the word *pericarditis*, one can come up with a simple definition of "inflammation surrounding the heart." The linking or combining vowel, which is *o* or *a*, links the root to the suffix or to another root. The combining vowel has no meaning of its own, it only joins parts of words. For example, in the term *hematology*, *hemat* means "blood" and *–logy* means the "study of," and the *o* links the two parts making the term mean the "study of blood."[11]

Pronunciation of medical terms can cause another barrier to searching for information. Often, when a patient hears a doctor discuss a particular symptom or condition, it is difficult to spell the word when doing research in a library or on the Internet. As we all know, one misspelled word when searching on a computer and, most likely, the search will turn up nothing. Miriam G. Austrin maps out a wonderful pronunciation chart as listed below:[12]

- *ch* Sometimes pronounced like *k*—example: chronic
- *ps* Pronounced like *s*—example: psychiatry
- *pn* Pronounced with only the *n*—example: pneumonia
- *c* and *g* Given soft sounds of *s* and *j*, respectively, before *e*, *i*, and *y*—examples: generic, giant, cycle, cytoplasm
- *ae* and *oe* Pronounced as *ee*—example: fasciae, coelom
- *i* Pronounced *eye* at the end of a word to form a plural—example: alveoli, glomeruli, fasciculi
- *es* Often pronounced as a separate syllable—example: nares (nah´reez)

Medical Thesauri

Since medical terminology can be so cumbersome, a number of standardized

---

11. Chabner, Davi-Ellen. *The Language of Medicine.* Philadelphia: W. B. Saunders, 1996. p. 3.
12. Austrin, Miriam G. and Harvey R. Austrin. *Learning Medical Terminology: A Worktext.* St. Louis, Mo.: Mosby Lifeline, 1995. p. 4.

thesauri have been developed. *MeSH*, or *Medical Subject Headings*, is the National Library of Medicine's (NLM) controlled vocabulary used for indexing articles, cataloging books and other holdings, and for searching major databases such as PubMed MEDLINE. *MeSH* terminology provides a consistent way to retrieve information that may use different terminology for the same concepts. The MeSH Browser (*www.ncbi.nlm.nih.gov:80/entrez/ meshbrowser.cgi*) may be used to find medical terms of interest and to see them in relationship to other terms. The terms appear in a hierarchy of related terms and each record includes scope notes, annotations, history notes, and allowable subheadings. The *MeSH* vocabulary is continually updated by subject specialists in various areas. Each year hundreds of new concepts are added and thousands of modifications are made; *2000 MeSH* includes more than 19,000 main headings, 110,000 Supplementary Concept (chemical) Records, and an entry vocabulary of over 300,000 terms.

NLM also developed the more comprehensive UMLS (Unified Medical Language System) Metathesaurus (*www.nlm.nih.gov/research/umls/*), which contains information about medical concepts and terms from many controlled vocabularies and classifications used in patient records, administrative health data, bibliographic and full-text databases, and expert systems. The *Metathesaurus* is organized by concept or meaning. Alternate names for the same concept (synonyms, lexical variants, and translations) are linked together. The 2000 edition of the *Metathesaurus* includes more than 730,000 concepts and 1.5 million concept names from over 50 different biomedical vocabularies, some in multiple languages. NLM does not charge for the *Metathesaurus*, but users must sign a "License Agreement for the Use of UMLS Products" found at *www.nlm.nih.gov/research/umls/license.html*.

CINAHL (Cumulative Index to Nursing and Allied Health Literature) began in the late 1940s when three librarians in Los Angeles indexed current nursing journals in the English language on three-by-five-inch cards. By 1961 the demand for an index to nursing journal literature resulted in the first printed version of the *Cumulative Index to Nursing Literature*. To keep pace with the trend toward a multidisciplinary approach to health care, the scope of coverage was expanded in 1977 to include allied health journals, thus changing the name to *CINAHL*. The *CINAHL Subject Heading List* contains over 10,600 terms and accepts the NLM's *MeSH* as the standard vocabulary for disease, drug, anatomical, and physiological concepts. The 2000 index also includes a revision of alternative therapies section. *CINAHL*, updated annually, is available in book index form or by subscribing to the *CINAHL* database through a vendor such as Ovid.[13]

---

13. *CINAHL 2000 Subject Heading List*. Glendale, Calif.: Cinahl Information Systems, 2000. pp. viii–x.

Pharmaceuticals

Drugs, chemical or biological substances used in the prevention or treatment of disease, offer additional problems for those looking for consumer health information. Each drug can potentially have three different names:

- **Generic (or official) name.** The generic (or official) name is the one recognized as identifying the drug for legal and scientific purposes. The generic name becomes public property after 17 years of use by the original manufacturer, and any drug manufacturer may use it after that time period. There is only one generic name for each drug.
- **Brand name.** The brand name of a drug is the private property of the individual drug manufacturer, and no competitor may use it. Brand names often have the superscript ® after the name, indicating it is a registered trade name.
- **Chemical name.** The chemical name is the drug's chemical formula, which is often long and complicated. Few consumers would use this formula; it is mostly used by chemists since it shows the structure of the drug.[14]

Drugs are administered in a variety of ways, as illustrated by Chabner below:[15]

Oral Administration: Drugs are given by mouth and are slowly absorbed into the bloodstream through the stomach or intestinal wall.

Sublingual Administration: Drugs are not swallowed but are placed under the tongue and allowed to dissolve in the saliva.

Rectal Administration. Suppositories (cone-shaped objects containing drugs) are inserted into the rectum.

Parenteral Administration: Drugs are administered by injection from a syringe through a hollow needle placed under the skin, into a muscle, vein, or body cavity.

Inhalation: Vapors or gases are taken into the nose or mouth and are absorbed into the bloodstream through the thin walls of the air sacs in the lungs.

Topical Application: Drugs are applied or rubbed into the skin or mucous membranes of the body.

Finally, there are many classes of drugs, as listed below:[16]

---

14. Chabner, pp. 748–750.
15. *Ibid.*, pp. 750–751.
16. *Ibid.*, pp. 752–758.

Analgesics: Drugs to relieve pain. Mild analgesics are used for mild to moderate pain, such as that caused by a headache or toothache. More potent analgesics are narcotics or opiods, which induce stupor; these drugs are only used to relieve severe pain because they can become habit forming.

Anesthetics: Agents that reduce or eliminate sensation—in the whole body (general anesthetic) or in a particular region (local anesthetic). General anesthetics are used for surgical procedures and depress the activity of the central nervous system, producing a loss of consciousness. Local anesthetics inhibit the conduction of impulses in sensory nerves in a region in which they are injected or applied.

Antibiotics: Chemical substances produced by a microorganism (bacterium, yeast, or mold) that inhibits or stops the growth of bacteria, fungi, or parasites. The use of antibiotics (penicillin was first used in 1945) has largely controlled many diseases, such as pneumonia and rheumatic fever.

Anticoagulants: A type of drug that prevents the clotting of blood. These drugs are used to prevent the formation of clots or to break up clots in blood vessels. They are also used to prevent coagulation in preserved blood used for transfusions.

Anticonvulsants: Drugs to prevent or reduce the severity of convulsions in various types of epilepsy.

Antidepressants: Drugs that treat the symptoms of depression by elevating mood, increasing physical activity and mental alertness, and improving appetite and sleep patterns.

Antidiabetics: Drugs used to treat diabetes mellitus. Patients with insulin-dependent (Type I) diabetes must receive daily injections of insulin. Patients with non-insulin-dependent (Type II) diabetes are given oral antidiabetic drugs that stimulate the production and release of insulin by the pancreas.

Antihistamines: Drugs that block the action of histamine, which is normally released in the body in allergic reactions and causes allergic symptoms such as hives, bronchial asthma, and hay fever. Antihistamines cannot cure the allergic reaction, but they can relieve the symptoms temporarily.

Cardiovascular Drugs: Drugs that act on the heart or the blood by increasing the force and efficiency of the heartbeat, correcting abnormal heart rhythms, and preventing angina (chest pain due to insufficient oxygen reaching the heart muscle).

Endocrine Drugs: Drugs used for male (androgens) and female (estrogens) hormone replacements. They are used to treat prostate cancer, endometriosis, breast cancer, and symptoms associated with menopause.

Gastrointestinal Drugs: Drugs used to relieve uncomfortable and potentially dangerous symptoms. Such drugs include antacids, antiulcer drugs, antidiarrheal drugs, and laxatives.

Respiratory Drugs: Drugs prescribed for the treatment of emphysema, asthma, and respiratory infections, such as pneumonia and bronchitis.

Sedatives: Drugs that relax and calm nervousness by depressing the central nervous system (brain), causing reduced mental activity.

Stimulants: Drugs that act on the brain to speed up vital processes (heart and respiration) in cases of shock and collapse.

Tranquilizers: Drugs used in controlling anxiety.

2
Understanding Consumer Health Concerns

The purpose of this chapter is to introduce readers to some of the major health concerns people currently face. This list is by no means comprehensive, yet it is reflective of common questions fielded by librarians in medical and public libraries. This list of major health concerns is based on the results of a 1998 poll that the Houston Academy of Medicine–Texas Medical Center conducted among libraries and health agencies in the Houston/Harris County, Texas, area to determine what health issues were of most concern to both library patrons and clients of health agencies.

Acquired Immune Deficiency Syndrome (AIDS)

According to the American Society of Clinical Pathologists (ASCP), AIDS is a fatal disease caused by a virus, a tiny organism similar to those that cause colds and flu. The virus that causes AIDS is the human immune deficiency virus (HIV). HIV infection causes people to get AIDS by damaging their immune systems. The immune system is what defends people against the many different organisms that can enter the body and cause sickness. Without the ability to resist disease, people with AIDS fall ill easily, get sick often, and have great difficulty recovering. People do not die from HIV infection directly. Rather, they die from the "opportunistic" infections and diseases they get because their immune system is not working.

The first cases of AIDS in the United States were documented in San Francisco by the Centers for Disease Control and Prevention (CDC) in the spring of 1981. As additional cases were reported in New York City and Los Angeles, the epidemic quickly became part of the world culture. Most people with AIDS (PWA) can lead active lives for a long time after diagnosis. Many, once they are debilitated by the disease, opt to live at home and be cared for by a family member. Because of this situation, many people can be affected by someone else's diagnosis. Both medical and public librarians can be approached by the PWA or by the caregiver. When working with either the PWA or the caregiver, it is important for the librarian to keep in mind that there are still stigmas associated with the disease and thus discretion is important.

For more information on AIDS see either **HAIL** (*www.hailinfo.org*) or **HIV InSite** (*http://hivinsite.ucsf.edu*).

Alzheimer's Disease

An estimated four million people in the United States suffer from Alzheimer's disease (AD). The disease usually begins after age 65, and risk of AD goes up with age. While younger people also may have AD, it is much less common. The National Institute on Aging reports that Alzheimer's disease (AD) is the most common cause of dementia in older people. A dementia is a medical condition that disrupts the way the brain works. AD affects the parts of the brain that control thought, memory, and language. Every day scientists learn more about AD, but right now the cause of the disease still is unknown and there is no cure.

AD begins slowly. Often the first symptom may be mild forgetfulness. People with AD may have trouble remembering recent events, activities, or the names of familiar people or things. Simple math problems may become hard to solve. Such difficulties may be a bother, but usually they are not serious enough to cause alarm. However, as the disease goes on, symptoms are more easily noticed and become serious enough to cause people with AD or their family members to seek medical help. For example, people with AD may forget how to do simple tasks, like brushing their teeth or combing their hair. They can no longer think clearly, and they begin to have problems speaking, understanding, reading, or writing. Later on, people with AD may become anxious or aggressive or wander away from home. Eventually, patients might need total care.

Doctors at specialized centers can diagnose probable AD correctly 80 to 90 percent of the time. They make this diagnosis by finding out more about the person's symptoms. The doctor may need some of the following information to make a diagnosis:

- complete medical history,
- basic medical tests of blood and urine to help the doctor eliminate other possible diseases,
- brain scans (computerized tomography, magnetic resonance imaging, or positron emission tomography) to see if anything looks abnormal,
- neuropsychological tests of memory, problem solving, attention, counting, and language.

No treatment can stop AD, but for some people in the early and middle stages of the disease certain drugs may alleviate some cognitive symptoms. Also, some medicines may help control behavioral symptoms of AD, such as sleeplessness, agitation, wandering, anxiety, and depression. Treating these symptoms often makes patients more comfortable and makes their care easier for caregivers. Scientists are testing new drugs for AD at many large teaching hospitals and universities. Some of these drugs have shown promise in easing symptoms in some patients. Most often, spouses or other family members provide the day-to-day care for people with AD. As the disease gets worse, people often need more and more care. This can be hard for caregivers and can affect their physical and mental health, family life, jobs, and finances.

For more information on AD, see **Alzheimer's Association** *(www.alz.org)*.

Asthma

According to the American Lung Association, more than 17 million Americans suffer from asthma, which is the seventh-ranking chronic condition in America. Asthma can be a life-threatening disease if not properly managed. People with asthma have very sensitive airways. Everyday things that cause little or no trouble for most people serve as asthma triggers for some people, leaving them gasping for breath. These triggers include:

- indoor and outdoor molds,
- animal dander (flakes from the skin, hair, or feathers of many pets, including dogs, cats, birds, rodents, and horses),
- dust mite particles (from microscopic insects present in house dust),
- cockroach particles,
- some foods or food additives,
- certain medications,
- and pollens from a variety of trees, weeds, and grasses.

These triggers, also known as allergens, affect the lungs. Less commonly, someone with allergies may develop asthma symptoms when an allergen is swallowed.

The most common symptoms of asthma are recurrent wheezing (a whistling or hissing sound as you breathe out), recurrent shortness of breath, recurrent feeling of tightness in the chest, or a cough that lasts for more than a week. Not all people with asthma wheeze. For some, coughing during the night or after exercise may be the main symptom. The American Medical Association reports that the key to controlling asthma is knowing how to spot the early warning signs of an asthma episode, which include:

- a chronic cough, especially at night;
- difficult or fast breathing;
- a feeling of chest tightness or discomfort;
- constant chest mucus; becoming out of breath more easily than usual;
- wheezing;
- fatigue;
- itchy, watery, or glassy eyes;
- an itchy, scratchy, or sore throat;

- a tendency to rub or stroke one's throat;
- sneezing;
- feeling that one's head is stopped up;
- headache;
- fever;
- restlessness;
- a runny nose;
- a change in the color of the face;
- or dark circles under the eyes.

Treatment is enhanced by knowing the warning signs and taking the correct amounts of medication prescribed by a doctor. Another treatment plan is to control the environment by eliminating the antigens that trigger an asthma attack.

For more information, see the Asthma section of **American Lung Association** (*www.lungusa.org/asthma*).

Breast Cancer

The National Cancer Institute reports that, after skin cancer, breast cancer is the most common type of cancer among women in the United States. Each year more than 180,000 women in this country learn they have breast cancer. The most common type of breast cancer begins in the lining of the ducts and is called ductal carcinoma. Another type, called lobular carcinoma, arises in the lobules. When breast cancer spreads outside the breast, cancer cells are often found in the lymph nodes under the arm. If the cancer has reached these nodes, it may mean that cancer cells have spread to other parts of the body (other lymph nodes and other organs, such as the liver or lungs) through the lymphatic system or the bloodstream. When breast cancer spreads, it is called metastatic breast cancer even though the secondary tumor is in another organ.

The risk of breast cancer increases gradually as a woman gets older. This disease is uncommon in women under the age of 35, but women age 40 and older are at risk. Most breast cancers occur in women over the age of 50, and the risk is especially high for women over age 60. Research has shown that the following conditions increase the risk for breast cancer:

- personal or family history of breast cancer,
- certain breast changes,
- breast density,
- exposure to radiation therapy,
- late childbearing,
- early menstruation (before age 12),

- late menopause (after age 55),
- never having children,
- or extended use of birth control pills.

Each of these factors increases the amount of time a woman's body is exposed to estrogen. The longer this exposure, the more likely she is to develop breast cancer. In most cases, doctors cannot explain why a woman develops breast cancer.

When breast cancer is found and treated early, the chances for survival are better. Women can take an active part in the early detection of breast cancer by having regular mammograms and clinical breast exams (breast exams performed by health professionals). Some women also perform breast self-exams. A screening mammogram is the best tool available for finding breast cancer early, before symptoms appear. A mammogram is a special kind of x-ray, which is used to look for breast changes in women who have no signs of breast cancer. Mammograms can often detect breast cancer before it can be felt, but can miss some cancers that are present or may find things that turn out not to be cancer. Detecting a tumor early does not guarantee that a woman's life will be saved, since some fast-growing cancers may already have spread to other parts of the body before being detected.

See **The Breast Clinic** (*www.thebreastclinic.com*) or **American Cancer Society** (*www.cancer.org*) for more information about breast cancer.

Diabetes

The National Institute of Diabetes and Digestive and Kidney Diseases reports that an estimated 16 million people in the United States have diabetes mellitus. About half of these people do not know they have diabetes and are not under care for the disorder. Each year about 798,000 people are diagnosed with diabetes. Although diabetes occurs most often in older adults, it is one of the most common chronic disorders in children in the United States. About 123,000 children and teenagers age 19 and younger have diabetes.

Diabetes is a disorder of metabolism, which is the way our bodies use digested food for growth and energy. Most of the food we eat is broken down by the digestive juices into a simple sugar called glucose. Glucose is the main source of fuel for the body. After digestion, the glucose passes into our bloodstream where it is available for body cells to use for growth and energy. For the glucose to get into the cells, insulin must be present. Insulin is a hormone produced by the pancreas, a large gland behind the stomach. When we eat, the pancreas should automatically produce the right amount of insulin to move the glucose from our blood into our cells. In people with diabetes, however, the pancreas either produces little or no insulin or the body cells do not respond to the insulin that is produced. As a result, glucose builds up in the blood, overflows into the urine, and passes out of the body. Thus the body loses its main source of fuel even though the blood contains large amounts of glucose.

There are three main types of diabetes:

- **Type 1 diabetes.** Once known as insulin-dependent diabetes mellitus, Type 1 diabetes is considered an autoimmune disease. When an autoimmune disease is present, the body's system for fighting infection (the immune system) turns against a part of the body. In Type 1 diabetes the immune system attacks the insulin-producing beta cells in the pancreas and destroys them. The pancreas then produces little or no insulin. Someone with Type 1 diabetes needs daily injections of insulin to live. Type 1 diabetes accounts for about 5 to 10 percent of diagnosed diabetes in the United States. Symptoms include increased thirst and urination, constant hunger, weight loss, blurred vision, and extreme tiredness. If not diagnosed and treated with insulin, a person can lapse into a life-threatening coma.
- **Type 2 diabetes.** The most common form of diabetes is Type 2 diabetes, which was once known as non-insulin-dependent diabetes mellitus. About 90 to 95 percent of people with diabetes have Type 2 diabetes. This form of diabetes usually develops in adults over the age of 40 and is most common among adults over age 55. About 80 percent of people with Type 2 diabetes are overweight. In Type 2 diabetes the pancreas usually produces insulin, but for some reason the body cannot use the insulin effectively. The end result is the same as for Type 1 diabetes—an unhealthy buildup of glucose in the blood and an inability of the body to make efficient use of its main source of fuel. The symptoms of Type 2 diabetes develop gradually and are not as noticeable as in Type 1 diabetes. Symptoms include feeling tired or ill, frequent urination (especially at night), unusual thirst, weight loss, blurred vision, frequent infections, and slow healing of sores.
- **Gestational diabetes.** Gestational diabetes develops or is discovered during pregnancy. This type usually disappears when the pregnancy is over, but women who have had gestational diabetes have a greater risk of developing Type 2 diabetes later in life.

See **American Diabetes Association** (*www.diabetes.org*) for more information on diabetes.

Heart Disease

According to the American Heart Association over 60 million Americans have one or more of the many types of heart and blood vessel diseases. In 1993 more than 950,000 people died from heart disease, accounting for over 42 percent of all deaths in the United States. Heart disease and blood vessel problems develop over time, as arteries that supply the heart or brain with blood slowly become clogged from a buildup of cells, fat, and cholesterol. This buildup is called plaque. When the blood flow gets blocked, a heart attack or stroke can occur.

There are five types of heart disease:

- **Hardening of the arteries,** or atherosclerosis, occurs when the inner walls of arteries become narrower due to a buildup of plaque. Blood clots form, so less blood can get through.
- **High blood pressure,** or hypertension, occurs when the pressure in the arteries is consistently above the normal range. Blood pressure is the force of blood pushing against blood vessel walls. The great danger is that people usually cannot tell they have high blood pressure. There are no signs, and therefore, the condition must be diagnosed by a doctor.
- **Heart attacks** occur when the blood flow to a part of the heart is blocked, often by a blood clot. If this clot cuts off the blood flow completely, the part of the heart muscle supplied by that artery begins to die. Symptoms of a heart attack include uncomfortable heavy feeling, pressure, pain, or squeezing in the center of the chest that lasts more than a few minutes; pain that goes to the shoulders, neck, or arms; and discomfort in the chest along with a light head, fainting, sweating, nausea, or shortness of breath.
- **Heart failure** occurs when the heart is not pumping blood as well as it should. The heart keeps working, but the body doesn't get all the blood and oxygen it needs. Signs of heart failure include swelling in the feet, ankles, and legs (called "edema"), and fluid buildup in the lungs (called "pulmonary congestion").
- **Stroke and transient ischemic attack (TIA),** or stroke warning, occur when a blood vessel that feeds the brain gets clogged or bursts. When that happens, that part of the brain cannot work and neither can the part of the body it controls. Major causes of stroke are uncontrolled high blood pressure, smoking, and heart disease. Warning signs include weak feeling in an arm, hand, or leg; lack of feeling on one side of the face or body; sudden lack of vision in one eye; speech difficulty; inability to understand what someone is saying; dizziness or loss of balance, and/or a sudden, very bad headache. (See the section "Stroke" later in this chapter.)

For more information about heart disease and stroke, see **American Heart Association** (*www.americanheart.com*).

Hepatitis

According to the National Institutes of Health, hepatitis consists of five distinct viruses that differ in mode of infection, length of viral incubation and pathogenicity, and the ability to produce a chronic disease that can progress to liver failure or cancer. All five forms of hepatitis can cause an acute illness.

- **Hepatitis A virus (HAV)** symptoms are often flu-like and include fever, fatigue, muscle and joint aches, as well as possible nausea, vomiting, and pain in the liver area. Recovery may take as long as a year. In about 10 percent of patients, acute HAV infection results in jaundice, but the risk of liver failure is very low, and there is no risk of the disease becoming chronic. Recovery is associated with lifelong immunity. The virus is spread by eating contaminated food or drinking contaminated water or ice cubes, by close personal contact such as kissing, or by sharing dirty needles.

- **Hepatitis B virus (HBV)** is either transient, lasting four to eight weeks, or is chronic. In 90 percent of infected people, acute infection produces symptoms that mimic flu, including fever, headache, muscle ache, and fatigue. About 15 to 20 percent of patients develop short-term arthritis-like problems. In 10 percent of patients, acute infection can result in jaundice. In acute hepatitis with jaundice, the risk of liver failure is about 1 in 100. Patients with chronic active HBV infection have a high risk of developing cirrhosis. Antibodies can neutralize the HB virus, preventing infection. The antigen has been used as a vaccine since 1975 and became generally available in 1982. Between 1 million and 1.5 million people die each year of HBV infection, making it one of the major causes of morbidity and death worldwide. The virus is most commonly transmitted by shared needles, by high-risk sexual behavior, from a mother to her newborn, and in the healthcare setting. For example, dentists, oral hygienists, and oral surgeons who are routinely exposed to blood on the job are at the top of the list for contracting HBV.

- **Hepatitis C virus (HCV)** is mostly characterized by jaundice. Cirrhosis develops in 10 to 20 percent of patients. The delay from initial infection to the development of cirrhosis usually is 10 to 30 years but sometimes is shorter (5 to 10 years). With the advent of new tests to screen blood donors, a very small percentage of the people who recently contracted HCV became infected through blood transfusions. HCV appears to be spread mainly through unprotected sexual contact, shared needles, untested blood products, and healthcare workers, although the method of infection is unknown in many cases. HCV is the most common form of chronic viral hepatitis in the United States and appears to be a major factor in the 25,000 deaths each year that are caused by chronic liver disease.

- **Hepatitis D virus (HDV),** or delta hepatitis, is the severest form of viral hepatitis, leading to cirrhosis in up to 70 percent of cases, often within a few years of the onset of disease. It accounts for less than 5 percent of the cases of chronic hepatitis. HDV occurs only in patients who have acute or chronic HBV hepatitis. Vaccine protection against HBV also serves against HDV.
- **Hepatitis E virus (HEV)** is an epidemic form of hepatitis that shares some characteristics with HAV, such as a lack of a chronic phase, and is present primarily in underdeveloped countries with contaminated water supplies. Outbreaks have not been observed in the United States, but at least 20 epidemics have occurred in 17 other countries.

There are no proven treatments for acute viral hepatitis except bed rest, a healthy diet, and avoidance of alcoholic beverages. Most patients experience complete recovery with restoration of liver function and clearance of the virus. Recent breakthroughs in understanding hepatitis B make the future therapy of this disease promising. The best approach to the control and prevention of hepatitis is vaccination of susceptible populations with HBV vaccine and, under special circumstances, with HAV vaccine.

An informative hepatitis Web site is maintained by the Centers for Disease Control and Prevention at *www.cdc.gov/ncidod/diseases/hepatitis/*.

High Blood Pressure

The National Heart, Lung, and Blood Institute reports that as many as 50 million Americans have high blood pressure, or hypertension, which is the medical term. Often known as the "Silent Killer," high blood pressure affects millions of people who do not know they have the disease. When high blood pressure is not detected and treated it can cause side effects that play a role in about 700,000 deaths a year from stroke, heart, and kidney disease.

To understand high blood pressure, one must first understand the basics of blood pressure itself. Blood is carried from the heart to all of the body's tissues and organs in vessels called arteries. Blood pressure is the force of the blood pushing against the walls of those arteries. Each time the heart beats (about 60 to 70 times a minute at rest), it pumps out blood into the arteries. Blood pressure is at its greatest when the heart contracts and is pumping the blood. This is called systolic pressure. When the heart is at rest, in between beats, blood pressure falls. This is the diastolic pressure. Blood pressure is always given as these two numbers. Usually they are written one above or before the other, such as 120/80, with the top or first number being the systolic and the bottom or second the diastolic.

Blood pressure tests are easy, and are usually taken in a doctor's office during an exam. Using a device called a sphygmomanometer, a healthcare professional takes blood pressure by placing a blood pressure cuff around an arm and inflating the cuff with air until blood circulation in the artery is temporarily stopped. A valve in the sphygmomanometer is opened and some of the air is slowly let out from the cuff, allowing the blood flow to start again. Using a stethoscope, the doctor or nurse listens to the blood flow in an artery at the inner elbow. The first sound heard is the heart as it pumps. This is the systolic pressure. More air is slowly released from the cuff. When the beating sound is no longer heard, the heart is at rest. This is the diastolic pressure.

High blood pressure can be treated in many ways, but mostly by a change of lifestyle and/or habits. People with high blood pressure are encouraged to lose weight, exercise, eat foods low in salt and sodium, limit alcohol intake, and regularly take high blood pressure medication.

Information about high blood pressure can be found on the American Heart Association's Web site (*www.americanheart.org/hbp*).

Influenza

Influenza, commonly called "the flu," is an infection of the respiratory tract caused by the influenza virus. According to the Centers for Disease Control and Prevention, compared with most other viral respiratory infections, such as the common cold, influenza infection often causes a more severe illness. Typical influenza illness includes fever (usually 100° to 103° Fahrenheit in adults and often higher in children), respiratory symptoms (such as cough, sore throat, runny or stuffy nose), headache, muscle aches, and often extreme fatigue. Although nausea, vomiting, and diarrhea can sometimes accompany influenza infection, especially in children, these symptoms are rarely the primary symptoms. The term "stomach flu" is a misnomer that is sometimes used to describe gastrointestinal illnesses caused by organisms other than influenza viruses. Most people who get the flu recover completely in one to two weeks, but some people develop serious and potentially life-threatening medical complications, such as pneumonia. In an average year, influenza is associated with more than 20,000 deaths nationwide and more than 100,000 hospitalizations. (The infamous 1918 influenza pandemic killed some 25 million people in a single year.) Flu-related complications can occur at any age; however, the elderly and people with chronic health problems are much more likely to develop serious complications after influenza infection than are younger, healthier people.

Flu vaccines are readily available each fall, and the American Medical Association recommends that the following high-risk groups receive a flu shot each year:

- People who are 50 years of age or older
- People who live in long-term care facilities (like nursing homes) who have chronic medical conditions

- People who have a health problem, such as asthma, diabetes, or heart, lung, or kidney disease
- People who have weakened immune systems, such as people living with HIV/AIDS or other disorders of the immune system, people receiving long-term treatment with certain drugs that affect the immune system, and people receiving cancer treatment with radiation or drugs that affect the immune system
- Anyone who is 6 months to 18 years of age and is receiving long-term treatment with aspirin (because these individuals could develop Reyes syndrome if they catch influenza)
- Women who will be past the third month of their pregnancy during the influenza season (in the United States the influenza season is roughly November through April)
- Healthcare workers and others (such as doctors, nurses, or their family members) who may come into close contact with people at risk of having influenza

The Centers for Disease Control's Web site **Influenza Prevention and Control** (*www.cdc.gov/ncidod/diseases/flu/fluvirus.htm*) is a good source of flu information.

Liver Disease

Alcohol-induced liver disease (ALD) is a major cause of illness and death in the United States as reported by the National Institute on Alcohol Abuse and Alcoholism. Fatty liver, the most common form of ALD, is reversible with abstinence. More serious ALD includes alcoholic hepatitis, characterized by persistent inflammation of the liver, and cirrhosis, characterized by progressive scarring of liver tissue. Either condition can be fatal, and treatment options are limited. During the past five years, research has significantly increased the understanding of the mechanisms by which alcohol consumption damages the liver. Approximately 10 to 35 percent of heavy drinkers develop alcoholic hepatitis, and 10 to 20 percent develop cirrhosis. In the United States, cirrhosis is the seventh leading cause of death among young and middle-aged adults. Approximately 10,000 to 24,000 deaths from cirrhosis may be attributable to alcohol consumption each year.

Normal liver function is essential to life. Alcohol-induced liver damage disrupts the body's metabolism, eventually impairing the function of other organs. Most of the alcohol a person drinks is eventually broken down by the liver. Inflammation is the body's response to local tissue damage or infection. Long-term alcohol consumption prolongs the inflammatory process, leading to excessive production of free radicals, or liver damaging cells, which can destroy healthy liver tissue.

Susceptibility to ALD differs considerably among individuals, so that even among people drinking similar amounts of alcohol, only some develop cirrhosis. Understanding the mechanisms of these differences may help clinicians identify and treat patients at increased risk for advanced liver damage. Researchers are seeking genetic factors that may underlie this variability. Results of this research may provide the basis for future gene-based therapies. Additionally, women develop ALD after consuming lower levels of alcohol over a shorter period of time compared with men. In addition, women have a higher incidence of alcoholic hepatitis and a higher mortality rate from cirrhosis than men. Many patients with ALD are infected with hepatitis C virus (HCV), which causes a chronic, potentially fatal liver disease. The presence of HCV may increase a person's susceptibility to ALD and influence the severity of alcoholic cirrhosis.

Abstinence is the cornerstone of ALD therapy. With abstinence, fatty liver and alcoholic hepatitis are frequently reversible, and survival is improved among patients with ALD, including those with cirrhosis. For terminally ill patients, liver transplantation remains the only effective treatment.

See **American Liver Foundation** (*www.liverfoundation.org*) for information about ALD and other diseases of the liver.

Pneumonia

Pneumococcal disease is a serious infection caused by a bacterium called *Streptococcus pneumoniae*, or *pneumococcus*. According to the Centers for Disease Control and Prevention, each year in the United States about 500,000 cases of pneumococcal pneumonia are diagnosed. Additionally, about 40,000 people die annually of pneumococcal infections. In persons over the age of 65 years, up to 30 percent of those infected die as a result of the infection, even when the patient is treated with antibiotics. Pneumococcal infection is also common in infants and toddlers under the age of 2 years. The most common type of pneumococcal infection is pneumonia, which is an infection of one or more lobes of the lung. Pneumococcal meningitis is an extremely serious infection, affecting the lining of the brain. Serious side effects such as paralysis, blindness, deafness, and death can occur as a result of this infection. When the pneumococcus invades the bloodstream, an infection called "bacteremia" results.

The most common symptoms of pneumococcal pneumonia are sudden shaking chills, cough, and fever. These symptoms are accompanied by chest congestion, a headache, and greenish, yellowish, or blood-tinged ("rusty") sputum. Breathing may be rapid and painful with sharp chest pain. About 20 to 30 percent of patients with pneumococcal pneumonia develop pneumococcal bacteremia. In turn, this infection can result in extremely serious complications such as meningitis, pericarditis (infection of the lining of the heart), peritonitis (infection of the lining of the abdomen), arthritis (infection of one or more joints), or death.

There is a pneumococcal vaccine available. The Advisory Committee on Immunization Practices (ACIP), the official committee charged with making vaccine recommendations in the United States, recommends that all persons age 65 years and older receive pneumococcal vaccine, along with the following persons 2 years of age and older:

- Persons with chronic heart, lung, or liver disease
- Persons with diabetes
- Persons with immunologic disorders or those who are immuno-compromised (cancer patients, persons with HIV infection, organ transplants, and those receiving steroids, chemotherapy, or radiation therapy)
- Persons who have had their spleen removed or have dysfunction of the spleen due to sickle cell anemia
- Persons who have a leakage of spinal fluid, or nephrotic syndrome (a chronic kidney condition that causes loss of protein through the urine)
- Persons with organ or bone marrow transplants
- Persons with chronic kidney failure

See the American Lung Association's Web site **Pneumonia** (*www.lungusa.org/ diseases/lungpneumoni.html*) for more information on pneumonia.

Prostate Cancer

After skin cancer, prostate cancer is the most commonly diagnosed form of cancer among men in the United States and is second only to lung cancer as a cause of cancer-related death among men. The American Cancer Society (ACS) estimates that 180,400 new cases of prostate cancer will be diagnosed and that approximately 31,900 men will die of the disease in 2000. At all ages, African American men are diagnosed with prostate cancer at later stages and die of the disease at higher rates than white men. The incidence of prostate cancer among African American men is the highest known rate in the world. According to the National Center for Chronic Disease Prevention and Health of the CDC, prostate cancer is most common among men age 65 years or older. About 80 percent of all men with clinically diagnosed cases of prostate cancer are in this age group. Because prostate cancer usually occurs at an age when other medical conditions, such as heart disease and stroke, may contribute significantly to the cause of death, the actual number of men who die with prostate cancer is unknown.

Two commonly used methods for detecting prostate cancer are currently available:

- **Digital rectal examination (DRE)** has been used for years as a screening test for prostate cancer. However, its ability to detect prostate cancer is limited. Small tumors often form in portions of the prostate that cannot be reached by a DRE. Doctors may also have difficulty distinguishing between benign abnormalities and prostate cancer, and the interpretation and results of the examination may vary with the experience of the examiner.

- **The prostate-specific antigen (PSA) measurement** is a blood test that many doctors use, but medical consensus on its use and interpretation has not been reached. PSA is an enzyme measured in the blood that may rise naturally as men age. It also rises in the presence of prostate abnormalities. However, the PSA test cannot distinguish prostate cancer from benign growth of the prostate and other conditions of the prostate, such as prostatitis. PSA testing also fails to detect some prostate cancers—about 20 percent of patients with biopsy-proven prostate cancer have PSA levels within normal range.

Physicians have become increasingly aware of the psychosocial aspects of prostate cancer and its treatment. Health professionals are realizing that the question is not merely how a life can be saved, but also how quality of life can be preserved. Many community education and support programs are available to help men and their families make informed decisions that will suit their needs, desires, and lifestyles. Appropriate treatment options for men with prostate cancer are based on the stage of the cancer at the time of diagnosis. Patient outcomes and the quality of life after treatment are influenced by the patient's age, the presence of other medical conditions, and the aggressiveness of the tumor.

See **American Cancer Society** (*www.cancer.org*) for more information about prostate cancer.

Sexually Transmitted Diseases

Sexually transmitted diseases (STDs), once called venereal diseases, are among the most common infectious diseases in the United States today. According to the National Institute of Allergy and Infectious Diseases (NIAID), more than 20 STDs have now been identified, and they affect more than 13 million men and women in this country each year. The annual comprehensive cost of STDs in the United States is estimated to be well in excess of $10 billion.

Understanding the basic facts about STDs—the ways in which they are spread, their common symptoms, and how they can be treated—is the first step toward prevention. It is important to understand at least five key points about all STDs in this country today:

- **STDs affect men and women of all backgrounds and economic levels.** They are most prevalent among teenagers and young adults. Nearly two-thirds of all STDs occur in people younger than 25 years of age
- **The incidence of STDs is rising,** in part because in the last few decades young people have become sexually active earlier yet are marrying later. In addition, divorce is more common. The net result is that sexually active people today are more likely to have multiple sex partners during their lives and are potentially at risk for developing STDs.
- **Most of the time, STDs cause no symptoms, particularly in women.** When and if symptoms develop, they may be confused with those of other diseases not transmitted through sexual contact. Even when an STD causes no symptoms, however, a person who is infected may be able to pass the disease on to a sex partner. That is why many doctors recommend periodic testing or screening for people who have more than one sex partner.
- **Health problems caused by STDs tend to be more severe and more frequent for women than for men,** in part because the frequency of asymptomatic infection means that many women do not seek care until serious problems have developed.
- **When diagnosed and treated early, many STDs can be treated effectively.** Some infections have become resistant to the drugs used to treat them and now require newer types of antibiotics. Experts believe that having STDs other than AIDS increases one's risk for becoming infected with the AIDS virus.

There are many types of STDs, including chlamydial infection, genital herpes, genital or venereal warts, gonorrhea, syphilis, trichomoniasis, bacterial vaginosis, cytomegalovirus infections, scabies, and pubic lice.

See **ASHA: American Social Health Association** (*www.ashastd.org/*) for more information about STDs.

Stroke

A stroke occurs when the blood supply to part of the brain is suddenly interrupted or when a blood vessel in the brain bursts, spilling blood into the spaces surrounding brain cells. Brain cells die when they no longer receive oxygen and nutrients from the blood, or when they are damaged by sudden bleeding into or around the brain. Ischemia is the term used to describe the loss of oxygen and nutrients for brain cells when there is inadequate blood flow. When blood flow to the brain is interrupted, some brain cells die immediately, while others remain at risk for death. With timely treatment these cells can be saved.

Even though a stroke occurs in the unseen reaches of the brain, the symptoms of a stroke are easy to spot. They include numbness or weakness, especially on one side of the body; confusion or trouble speaking or understanding speech; trouble seeing in one or both eyes; trouble walking, dizziness, or loss of balance or coordination; or severe headache with no known cause. All of the symptoms of stroke appear suddenly, and often multiple symptoms appear at the same time. For this reason, stroke can usually be distinguished from other causes of dizziness or headache. When stroke symptoms appear, medical attention is needed immediately.

There are two forms of stroke: ischemic, which involves blockage of a blood vessel supplying the brain, and hemorrhagic, which involves bleeding into or around the brain. A transient ischemic attack (TIA), sometimes called a ministroke, starts just like a stroke but then resolves leaving no noticeable symptoms or deficits. The occurrence of a TIA is a warning that the person is at risk for a more serious and debilitating stroke. Recurrent stroke is a major contributor to stroke disability and death, with the risk of severe disability or death from stroke increasing with each stroke recurrence. The risk of a recurrent stroke is greatest right after a stroke, with the risk decreasing with time. About 3 percent of stroke patients will have another stroke within 30 days of their first stroke and one-third of recurrent strokes take place within two years of the first stroke.

Binswanger's disease, also affiliated with stroke, is a rare form of dementia characterized by cerebrovascular lesions in the deep white-matter of the brain, loss of memory and cognition, and mood changes. Patients usually show signs of abnormal blood pressure, stroke, blood abnormalities, disease of the large blood vessels in the neck, and disease of the heart valves. Other prominent features of the disease include urinary incontinence, difficulty walking, parkinsonian-like tremors, and depression. These symptoms, which tend to begin after the age of 60, are not always present in all patients and may sometimes appear only as a passing phase. Seizures may also be present. There is no specific course of treatment for Binswanger's disease. Treatment is symptomatic, often involving the use of medications to control high blood pressure, depression, heart arrhythmias, and low blood pressure.

According to the National Institute of Neurological Disorders and Stroke, some people are at a higher risk for stroke than others. Unmodifiable risk factors include age, gender, race/ethnicity, and stroke family history. In contrast, other risk factors for stroke, like high blood pressure or cigarette smoking, can be changed or controlled by the person at risk. Stroke strikes all age groups, from fetuses still in the womb to centenarians. It is true, however, that older people have a higher risk for stroke than the general population and that the risk for stroke increases with age. Gender also plays a role in risk for stroke. Men have a higher risk for stroke, but more women die from stroke. Stroke seems to run in some families. The most important risk factors for stroke are hypertension, heart disease, diabetes, and cigarette smoking. Others include heavy alcohol consumption, high blood cholesterol levels, illicit drug use, and genetic or congenital conditions, particularly vascular abnormalities.

For more information about stroke, see **American Heart Association** (*www.americanheart.org*).

Suicide

Suicide is a tragic and potentially preventable public health problem. According to the National Institute of Mental Health, in 1996, the most recent year for which statistics are available, suicide was the ninth leading cause of death in the United States. Specifically, 10.8 out of every 100,000 persons died by suicide. The total number of suicides was approximately 31,000, or 1.3 percent of all deaths, which was about the same number of deaths as from AIDS. It is estimated that there were 500,000 suicide attempts.

Suicidal behavior is complex. Some risk factors vary with age, gender, and ethnic group and may even change over time. The risk factors for suicide frequently occur in combination. Research has shown that 90 percent of people who kill themselves have depression or another diagnosable mental or substance abuse disorder. Adverse life events in combination with other strong risk factors, such as depression, may lead to suicide. However, suicide and suicidal behavior are not normal responses to the stresses experienced by most people. Many people experience one or more risk factors and are not suicidal. Other risk factors include prior suicide attempt, family history of mental or substance abuse disorder, family history of suicide, family violence (including physical or sexual abuse), firearms in the home, incarceration, and exposure to the suicidal behavior of others (including family members, peers, and/or via the media in news or fiction stories).

More than four times as many men than women die by suicide. However, women report attempting suicide about twice as often as men. Suicide by firearms is the most common method for both men and women, accounting for 59 percent of all suicides in 1996. Over the last several decades, the suicide rate in young people has increased dramatically. In 1996 suicide was the third leading cause of death in 15- to 24-year-olds—12.2 of every 100,000 persons—following unintentional injuries and homicide. Suicide was the fourth leading cause in 10- to 14-year-olds, with 298 deaths among 18.9 million children in this age group. For adolescents aged 15 to 19, there were 1,817 suicide deaths among 18.6 million adolescents.

Preventive interventions for suicide must be complex and intensive if they are to have lasting effects over time. Recognition and appropriate treatment of mental and substance abuse disorders for particular high-risk age, gender, and cultural groups is the most promising way to prevent suicide and suicidal behavior.

See **SpanUSA** (*www.spanusa.org*) for more information on suicide.

Tuberculosis

Tuberculosis (TB), a chronic bacterial infection, causes more deaths worldwide than any other infectious disease. TB is spread through the air and usually infects the lungs, although other organs are sometimes involved. Each year, eight million people worldwide develop active TB and three million die. According to the National Institute of Allergy and Infectious Diseases, TB has reemerged as a serious public health problem. In 1998 a total of 18,371 active TB cases in all 50 states and the District of Columbia were reported to the CDC. Minorities are affected disproportionately by TB. In 1995, 54 percent of active TB cases among African American and Hispanic people, with an additional 17.5 percent found in Asians. In some sectors of U.S. society, TB rates now surpass those in the world's poorest countries. Among African American men in New York City aged 35 to 44, for example, 315 out of 100,000 had active TB in 1993, many times the national average of 9.8 cases per 100,000.

TB is primarily an airborne disease that is not likely to be transmitted through personal items touched by those with TB. Adequate ventilation is the most important measure to prevent the transmission of TB, which occurs only after prolonged exposure to someone with active TB. People are most likely to be contagious when their sputum contains bacilli, when they cough frequently, and when the extent of their lung disease, as revealed by a chest x-ray, is great. TB is spread from person to person in microscopic germs expelled from the lungs when a TB sufferer coughs, sneezes, speaks, sings, or laughs. Only those with active TB are contagious.

With appropriate antibiotic therapy TB usually can be cured. In recent years, however, drug-resistant cases of TB have increased dramatically. Drug resistance results when patients fail to take their medicine consistently for the 6 to 12 months necessary to destroy all vestiges of tuberculosis. In some U.S. cities, more than 50 percent of patients—often homeless people, drug addicts, and others caught in poverty—fail to complete their prescribed course of TB therapy. One reason for this lack of compliance is that TB patients may feel better after only two to four weeks of treatment and stop taking their TB drugs, some of which can have unpleasant side effects.

TB is largely a preventable disease. In the United States, prevention has focused on identifying infected individuals early and treating them with drugs in a program of directly observed therapy.

The Centers for Disease Control and Prevention maintains an informative tuberculosis Web site at *www.cdc.gov/nchstp/tb/*.

3
Exploring Complementary and Alternative Medicine

According to the American Medical Association, if you have ever taken high-dose vitamins, used an herbal remedy, or sought treatment from a chiropractor, you are among the millions all over the world who use alternative medicine to ward off illness or treat ailments. Known by a variety of terms—complementary, holistic, unorthodox, integrative—alternative medicine refers to most treatment practices that are not considered conventional medicine (the type of medicine widely practiced or accepted by the mainstream medical community). Although the majority of medicine practiced in the United States is conventional, approximately 70 to 90 percent of health care worldwide is delivered by what would be considered an alternative tradition or practice. Incorporating hundreds of different philosophies and procedures, alternative therapies are usually ideologically based and often not backed by scientific research that measures safety or effectiveness. Some alternative therapies have dangerous side effects, and, often, people who use alternative therapies do so in place of conventional medical therapies, possibly jeopardizing their health.

Recent Growth of Complementary and Alternative Medicine

The November 11, 1998, issue of *JAMA*, which was dedicated to complementary and alternative medicine (CAM), reported that:

- Four out of ten Americans use some form of alternative medicine.
- Americans visited alternative therapy practitioners 629,000 times in 1997, a 47 percent increase over the 427,000 visits made in 1990.
- Americans spent approximately $27 billion out-of-pocket (not covered by insurance) on alternative therapies in 1997, which is about the same as the estimated 1997 out-of-pocket spending for all U.S. physician services.

A recent article published in the *Journal of Clinical Medicine* reports that 83 percent of patients surveyed at the University of Texas M. D. Anderson Cancer Center between December 1997 and June 1998 had used CAM, though the authors stressed that the M. D. Anderson patients often used alternative therapies in conjunction with traditional therapies managed by a physician.[1] In a similar study of breast cancer patients by researchers at the London Regional Cancer Center in Ontario, Canada, 66.7 percent of survey participants (a random sample of Ontario women diagnosed with breast cancer in 1994 or 1995) reported using alternative therapies, most often in an attempt to boost the immune system. CAM practitioners (chiropractors, herbalists, acupuncturists, traditional Chinese medicine practitioners, and/or naturopathic practitioners) were visited by 39.4 percent of the respondents, and 62 percent reported use of products such as vitamins/minerals, herbal medicines, green tea, and special foods.[2] According to an article published in *JAMA* in 1997, 75 medical schools included courses in CAM in their curriculum.[3]

Although many of the current alternative therapies have been around for centuries, it has been since the 1960s that the appeal of CAM has grown. In January 1993 there were two major events in the promotion of alternative medicine. First, a landmark article on alternative therapies by Dr. David Eisenberg was published in the *New England Journal of Medicine*;[4] second, the National Center for Complementary and Alternative Medicine was created at the National Institutes of Health.

Why has there been such an explosion in CAM in recent years? One reason might be a dissatisfaction with biomedicine that focuses on disease and its cure by surgery, drugs, and/or sophisticated technology. Additionally, contemporary medicine seems to concentrate on cure and not prevention, which can be much more cost effective. Many modern therapies and/or cures, such as chemotherapy, have been shown to have serious side effects or can be too expensive for patients, especially those who have no insurance. CAM enables individual patients to play an active role in their own health care. Having control over treatment puts people at ease and allows them to concentrate on getting well. Finally, perhaps this explosion is due to the enormous amount of publicity alternative medicine has received coupled with aggressive marketing. One must only watch the local television news, read the local newspaper, or peruse the latest health books to see the proliferation of material available.

---

1. Richardson, Mary Ann, et al. "Complementary/Alternative Medicine Use in a Comprehensive Cancer Center and the Implications for Oncology." *Journal of Clinical Oncology* 18, no. 13 (2000): p. 2505.

2. Boon, Heather, et al. "Use of Complementary/Alternative Medicine by Breast Cancer Survivors in Ontario: Prevalence and Perceptions." *Journal of Clinical Oncology* 18, no. 13 (2000): p. 2515.

3. Wetzel, M. W., et al. "Courses Involving Complementary and Alternative Medicine at US Medical Schools." *JAMA* 280, no. 9 (1998): p. 784.

4. Eisenberg, D. M., et al. "Unconventional Medicine in the United States: Prevalence, Costs, and Patterns of Use." *New England Journal of Medicine* 328, no. 28 (1993): pp. 246–252.

Another factor may be that modern physicians are too rushed and consequently do not spend enough time with patients, nor do they communicate effectively with them. This can leave the patient disenchanted with conventional medicine.

Major Types of Complementary and Alternative Medicine

There are three different types of CAM: hands-on therapies, mind-body therapies, and herbal healing and lifestyle approaches. There is a lot of overlap between the categories, and some techniques fall into more than one category.

Hands-On Therapies

Hands-on approaches all involve touching or manipulating the body, either with hands or physical objects and include such techniques as cracking bones, adjusting the spine, and rubbing sore spots. Hands-on therapies include acupuncture, chiropractic, osteopathy, and massage therapy.

Acupuncture: A treatment in which special needles are inserted into points just under the skin to help correct and rebalance the flow of energy, promoting pain relief and healing. The word acupuncture comes the Latin *acus*, for "needle," and *puntura*, "to puncture." This ancient Chinese therapy has been continuously refined over its 4,500-year history. Millions of people have used acupuncture for a variety of health conditions. The treatment is often used in conjunction with more conventional methods and has gained wide acceptance. Some of the conditions treated with acupuncture include nausea, pain, treatment of lung problems (such as asthma), rehabilitation from damage to the nervous system (such as that caused by a stroke), and treatment for addictions to alcohol, tobacco, and other drugs. Although the American Association of Medical Colleges reports that no medical school in the United States provides acupuncture training, some chiropractic schools have elective 200-hour programs. The American Holistic Medical Association has developed a 300-hour program for physicians. Several programs located throughout the country offer rigorous comprehensive preparation that takes as long as 36 months and includes a clinical residency with 500 hours of supervised clinical work before licensure is granted. The National Commission for the Certification of Acupuncturists offers a competency test that is used in some states.[5]

---

5. Wright, Kathleen Dredge. "Acupuncture." *Gale Encyclopedia of Medicine*. Detroit: Gale Research, 1999. p. 30.

Chiropractic: Introduced in 1885, chiropractic is based on the belief that the body's healing powers are centered in the central nervous system and run along the spine. When a nerve is interfered with, the organ(s) it serves will become damaged or diseased. The cure for illness, therefore, is to remove the stress on the nerves by manipulating the spine. Chiropractors carefully use their fingers to feel along the spine, looking for misaligned vertebrae, muscle tension, swelling, or other signs of spinal trouble. Chiropractic is perhaps the most widely accepted of the alternative therapies. Chiropractors are licensed by the various states, and, in many states, are allowed to admit patients to hospitals and treat them there. Many doctors will refer patients to chiropractors, and treatment is covered by many insurance plans.[6]

Osteopathy: A system and philosophy of health care that separated from traditional (allopathic) medical practice about a century ago, osteopathy concentrates on the musculoskeletal system in a manner that is similar to chiropractic. Osteopathy shares many of the same goals as traditional medicine, but places greater emphasis on the relationship between the organs and the musculoskeletal system as well as on treating the whole individual rather than just the disease. Like chiropractic, osteopathy presumes that energy flowing through the nervous system is influenced by the supporting structures that encase and protect it, the skull and the vertebral column. A defect in the musculoskeletal system is believed to alter the flow of this energy and cause disease. Correcting the defect cures the disease. Near the middle of the 20th century, the equivalence of medical education between osteopathy and allopathic medicine was recognized and the DO degree (Doctor of Osteopathy) was granted official parity with the MD (Doctor of Medicine) degree. As of 1998 osteopaths constituted 5.5 percent of American physicians, or approximately 45,000.[7]

Massage Therapy and Body Work: Any kind of systematic manipulation of the soft tissues of the body (i.e., muscle and connective tissue). Manipulation can consist of any combination of rubbing, kneading, slapping, tapping, rolling, pressing, or jostling employed to make the recipient feel better. Besides helping the recipient relax, soothing sore muscles, reducing some types of swelling, and improving general well being, massage therapy may also help with hypertension, burns, chronic pain (including from arthritis, backaches, and migraines), rashes and other skin conditions, addictions, depression, and the stress and pain of labor. There are many types of massage, including traditional European versions and contemporary Western massage. Other body

---

6. Fox, Arnold, and Barry Fox. *Alternative Healing*. Franklin Lakes, N.J.: Career Press, 1996. pp. 15–16.
7. Polsdorfer, J. Ricker. "Osteopathy." *Gale Encyclopedia of Medicine*. p. 2113.

work methods include acupressure and shiatsu, which are similar to acupuncture without needles.[8]

Mind-Body Therapies

Mind-body therapies are based on the belief that mental and emotional states can affect the body. The five kinds of mind-body therapies are relaxation techniques, meditation, hypnotherapy, biofeedback, and spiritual healing.

Relaxation Techniques: Many mind-body techniques are based on the premise that relaxation can help reduce the hazardous stress hormones in the body and possibly undo some of the damage. So can feeling in control of your body and health.[9] An example of a relaxation technique includes arranging a short period of time every day when you know you will not be disturbed; finding a comfortable sitting position, closing eyes, and breathing slowly; with each exhalation repeating a comforting word or phrase; banishing all distracting or judgmental thoughts; and opening eyes for the last minute or two but continuing to sit, repeating the focus word and breathing slowly.[10]

Meditation : One of the oldest and most widely practiced mind-body therapies, meditation originated as a spiritual practice within traditional religious contexts. The original goal was to lead the practitioner to a more absolute, unconditional, or sacred state of consciousness. There is, however, nothing inherently religious or spiritual about meditation, which can be taken from the traditional cultural or religious setting and used as a tool to improve health and quality of life. Meditation techniques all share a structured mental process that steadies and deepens awareness by bringing it to rest on a stable focus. This process may be accomplished by resting the attention on a physical sensation (such as breathing), a thought or word that is silently repeated, an external object (such as a candle's flame or a statue), or the process of attention itself. By intentionally directing and regulating attention, the mediator modifies the functioning of the mind and its relationship to the body.[11]

Hypnotherapy: Originally known as "mesmerism," hypnosis is an artificially induced state of intense concentration. Begun in the 1700s, by the mid–1800s hypnosis was being used to relieve pain and as an anesthetic for surgery. The American Medical Association has approved the use of hypnosis

8. Dillard, James, and Terra Ziporyn. *Alternative Medicine for Dummies: A Reference for the Rest of Us.* Foster City, Calif.: IDG Books Worldwide, 1998. pp. 166–167.
9. Dillard and Ziporyn, p. 40.
10. Dillard and Ziporyn, pp. 187–188.
11. Jonas, Wayne B., and Jeffrey S. Levin. *Essentials of Complementary and Alternative Medicine.* Philadelphia: Lippincott, Williams & Wilkins, 1999. p. 523.

since 1958, and currently over 15,000 physicians use hypnotherapy as an adjunct to their more traditional therapies. Many types of health professionals use hypnosis in their practices, but certified hypnotherapists specialize in hypnosis alone. Hypnotherapists speak to the "unconscious" mind, since the "conscious" mind tends to reject suggestions. The less-critical subconscious mind tends to accept what it is told as reality. Getting to the subconscious mind, it is reasoned, allows healers to implant healing suggestions where they will do the most good.[12]

Biofeedback: Biofeedback is the use of instrumentation to monitor, amplify, and feed back physiological information, so that a patient can learn to change or regulate the process being monitored. In biofeedback therapy, clinical goals are achieved through psychophysiological self-regulation, a term that accurately describes the process in which mental, emotional, and physiological strategies and skills are learned and used by the patient. The feedback of information assists the patient in gaining self-regulation and physiological control.[13]

Spiritual Healing: Going to regular religious services or just taking a "spiritual" approach to life may help prevent, and may even cure, some diseases. Even if it does not, having a hopeful, peaceful, contented attitude, which is how spirituality is defined, is a desirable way to go through life. Many forms of traditional medicine from around the world also rely largely on spiritual healing, which may, in part, explain why so many people are turning to Native American, Latin American, and Tibetan medicine for new ideas about health care. Many of these traditions include herbal remedies, massage therapies, and exotic rituals, but they all rest on a spiritual foundation.[14]

Herbal Healing and Lifestyle Approaches

The five types of herbal and lifestyle approaches are dietary supplements, herbs and botanicals, homeopathy, aromatherapy, and nutrition and diet.

Dietary Supplements: Traditionally, dietary supplements refer to products made of one or more of the essential nutrients, such as vitamins, minerals, and protein. The 1994 Dietary Supplement Health and Education Act (DSHEA) broadened the definition to include, with some exceptions, any product intended for ingestion as a supplement to the diet. This definition includes herbs, botanicals, and other plant-derived substances, amino acids, concentrates, metabolites, constituents, and extracts of these substances. DSHEA requires

---

12. Fox and Fox, p. 21.
13. Jonas and Levin, pp. 410–411.
14. Dillard and Ziporyn, pp. 300–301.

manufacturers to include the words "dietary supplement" on product labels. Dietary supplements come in many forms, including tablets, capsules, powders, softgels, gelcaps, and liquids. Though commonly associated with health food stores, dietary supplements also are sold in grocery, drug, and discount stores, as well as through mail-order catalogs, television programs, the Internet, and direct sales. The Food and Drug Administration oversees dietary supplement safety, manufacturing, and product information (for example, claims made on a product's labeling, package inserts, and accompanying literature). The Federal Trade Commission regulates the advertising of dietary supplements.[15]

Herbs and Botanicals: People have used plants and herbs to treat illness as long as they have been treating their ailments. Herbal remedies remain the main, and often the only, form of healing in much of the world. Many modern drugs are derived from plants, including aspirin (originally from willow bark and later from meadowsweet), reserpine (a blood pressure medicine and tranquilizer from Indian snakeroot), and morphine (from the opium poppy). Herbal remedies can be made from flowers, leaves, fruits, or whole parts of plants.[16]

Homeopathy: Homeopathy is a system of healing that uses diluted portions of natural substances to cure symptoms of disease, and the more diluted the better. Remedies aim at revving up an invisible "life force" or "vital energy" that, at first, actually stimulates symptoms. Homeopaths consider symptoms to be good at first because they are the body's way of healing itself. Homeopathy is based on "the hair of the dog" theory that you cure a problem with a little bit of the same thing that made you sick.[17]

Aromatherapy: Aromatherapy involves inhaling essential oils from plants or rubbing them into the skin. Essential oils, the stuff that makes the plants smell, are extracted from the plants and concentrated. Aromatherapists say that essential oils do more than just make you smell good. They lift your mood and affect virtually every system in your body, including circulation, hormone levels, heart rate, nervous system, and digestion. Some of the effects of aromatherapy—including alteration of brain waves, killing of germs, lowering of blood pressure, or reduction of inflammation—are due to the chemistry of the oils. Other effects are attributed to a spiritual power that helps balance body, mind, and spirit.[18]

Nutrition and Diet: Nutritional medicine involves therapeutic application of a dietary and nutritional modification to reestablish bodily harmony. Al-

---

15. *www.fda.gov/fdac/features/1998/598_guide.html*
16. Dillard and Ziporyn, pp. 221–222.
17. Dillard and Ziporyn, pp. 127–129.
18. Dillard and Ziporyn, pp. 239–240.

though there are specific types of diet therapy (such as the Macrobiotic, Pritikin, Waianae, and Gerson diets), nutritional medicine can be as simple as reducing salt intake for a person with high blood pressure or reducing sugar intake for a person with diabetes.[19]

19. Jonas and Levin, p. 490.

PART II

Consumer Health Resources for Libraries

4
Recommended Consumer Health Web Sites

This chapter serves as a guide to the very best Web sites for consumer health—we recommend them all. Each of the sites listed are also included as links just a double-click away on the CD-ROM that accompanies this book. Although we carefully examined nearly 400 sites to create this list, less than 100 were usefully informative enough to make the cut. We hope to have saved you some time and energy.

Criteria for Selecting Notable Web Sites

Content

To state the obvious, a Web site must provide consumer health content in order to be recommended. The three types of content a consumer health Web site can provide are:

- Original consumer health content
- Links to other consumer health information resources
- Online services for healthcare consumers (for example, online medical records, health calculators, "Ask-an-Expert" services)

The above types of content can have one or more of the following characteristics:

- Quantity
- Uniqueness
- Quality
- Navigability (good Web design)

To be selected on the basis of content, a site had to be notable in some combination of the above characteristics. For example, **MayoClinic.com** is notable for presenting a good quantity of high-quality, original content; **Yahoo! Health** offers no original content and exercises no quality control, yet the quantity of consumer health links provided makes it a notable site; **MEDLINE***plus* provides no original content and fewer links than **Yahoo! Health**, but the quality control and navigability of **MEDLINE***plus* make it notable; the **NORD** Web site makes the list because of the uniqueness of the information it provides.

Popularity

The authors also considered a site's popularity with healthcare consumers. Although it is true that popular sites do not always offer the best information, such sites are certainly notable. In the case of commercial consumer health Web sites, popularity was an especially important consideration, since so many Web sites of this type are all but identical when it comes to content.

What Was Left Off the List

There are four broad categories of material omitted from this list of Web sites:

- Since the audience for this book is composed mostly of English-speaking North Americans, the list is highly slanted towards English-language, North American Web sites.
- As it is impossible to know of all the consumer health sites on the Web, some notable consumer health Web sites were no doubt left off this list. It is our hope that suggestions made by readers of this book and by visitors to **Recommended Consumer Health Web Sites** will bring these overlooked Web sites to our attention.
- Potentially useful consumer health Web sites that exist principally to market specific services or products without providing additional consumer health information were left off the list. An example of such a site is the extremely popular **eDiets.com,** which markets the **eDiets.com** diet programs but otherwise offers little to those who have not enrolled in and paid for one of the **eDiets.com** programs.
- Finally, some deserving Web sites were left off the list because their consumer health content is best accessed through other Web sites. For example, the **National Institutes of Health** Web site was left off the list because its (extremely valuable) consumer health information is most easily accessed via **MEDLINE***plus* or **healthfinder.**

About the Annotations

Tables

The tables associated with each Web site listed below are more or less self-explanatory.

A "Yes" under "Privacy Policy" means that the Web site has a prominently displayed privacy policy; however, a "Yes" under this heading does not ensure the quality of that privacy policy. Users concerned about privacy need to read privacy policies carefully and must be aware that not all Web sites live up to the promises made in their privacy policies. On the other hand, the fact that a Web site does not have a prominently displayed privacy policy does not

Cookie Cutter Web Sites: Commercial Consumer Health on the Web

Mimesis is particularly rampant among the large, for-profit Web sites, as exemplified by such sites as **WebMD** and **drkoop.com**. In fact, the following features are common to just about every site in this genre:

- Consumer health information organized by area of interest or "community" (that is, "Men's Health," "Women's Health," "Senior Health")
- Consumer health information organized by disease and condition
- Free e-mail alerts on specific health topics
- Current health news
- A searchable drug-information database
- An online medical dictionary
- A "My HealthWeb site.com" feature that allows consumers to customize the Web site to feature the topics in which they are interested
- Chat and/or e-mail-based communities or support groups focused on specific medical conditions
- An "Ask a Doctor" (or other medical expert) feature which allows consumers to submit health questions to medical professionals via e-mail
- Health calculators that allow consumers to determine their ideal weight, ideal calorie intake, risk for heart disease, and so on
- Online medical records that allow consumers to store their health information on the Web site, and online journal services that allow consumers to maintain health journals on the Web site (raising considerable privacy issues)
- Online shopping services

It is unusual to find anything that varies from the above on for-profit consumer health Web sites. The fact that almost every commercial site offers the same information and services explains why so many have gone out of business or are on the brink of financial ruin. The hullabalooed **drkoop.com** (a.k.a. "drkoop.broke") has had financial problems since its inception, and the heavily advertised **mothernature.com** went out of business despite its blatant linking of information resources with online sales (i.e., articles praising the virtues of Vitamin X were laced with links that allowed consumers to purchase Vitamin X from the **mothernature.com** online store).

necessarily mean that it does not respect visitor privacy. (Oddly, the Web site of Alcoholics Anonymous does not have a privacy policy even though protecting the individual's privacy is a core value of AA.)

A "Yes" under "Advertisements" means that the Web site sells space to advertisers much as a magazine or commercial television station might. The more conscientious sites divulge their advertising policies and detail what lines, if any, are drawn between advertisers and editorial control of the site's content.

A "Yes" under "Direct Sales" means that the Web site sells products directly to consumers. In cases where a site sells only publications (such as books or videos), this is noted by the word "Publications." The more reputable sites make clear distinctions between the informational and online sales areas of their Web sites.

About

The "About" section of each annotation attempts to explain who, exactly, is behind the Web site and what their purpose is. Great care was taken in this area, as knowing who is behind a Web site and what motivates them is often the best way to evaluate the information found on that site.

Keep in mind that Web sites can change overnight. All of these sites were thoroughly evaluated as close to this book's publication date as possible. In a nutshell, anything that was true about Site X an hour ago may not be true now, and the only way to know for sure what is on Site X right at the moment is to visit it and see for yourself.

AARP

www.aarp.org

Type of Site	Privacy Policy	Advertisements	Direct Sales
Nonprofit	Yes	Yes	Yes

About: The American Association of Retired Persons (AARP) is a nonprofit organization "dedicated to shaping and enriching the experience of aging for our members and for all Americans." Anyone age 50 or older may join AARP, which currently claims some 30 million members. Among other activities, AARP lobbies Congress on health-related matters of interest to seniors (for example, Medicare, prescription drug benefits) and offers member services that include a group health insurance plan and a mail-order pharmacy.

Contents: The "Health & Wellness" section of **AARP** provides seniors with information in such areas as fitness, caregiving, nursing homes, and health insurance. Visitors to the site can participate in, and get support from "Wellness Discussions" and "Caregivers Circle."

Special Features: AARP is an especially good site for information on health insurance and healthcare costs as they relate to seniors.

Achoo

www.achoo.com

Type of Site	Privacy Policy	Advertisements	Direct Sales
Commercial	Yes	Yes	No

About: **Achoo** is owned and managed by MNI Systems Corporation, an Internet healthcare company based in Mississauga, Ontario, Canada.

Content: Covers a broad spectrum of health issues, including consumer health, clinical medicine, alternative medicine, and medical economics. **Achoo** links to other health-related Web sites, but only after **Achoo** editors have evaluated the sites for content, design, and maintenance.

Special Features: "Achoo News & Press" provides original content on a variety of health topics. Produced by Health Scout, most of these stories are careful about citing their sources of information.

ADA.org

www.ada.org

Type of Site	Privacy Policy	Advertisements	Direct Sales
Nonprofit	No	Yes	Yes

About: The American Dental Association (ADA) is the largest professional association of dentists in the United States. In part, ADA's mission "promotes the profession of dentistry by enhancing the integrity and ethics of the profession, strengthening the patient/dentist relationship and making membership a foundation of successful practice."

Content: The "Public" section of **ADA.org** includes such features as "Oral Health Topics A-Z," "ADA News Releases," and special sections for kids, parents, mature adults, and teachers.

Special Features: Consumers can search the "ADA Seal of Acceptance" section of **ADA.org** to identify oral-health products that the ADA has found to be safe and effective. The "Find a Dentist" feature allows consumers to search for ADA-member dentists by any combination of name, location, and specialty.

Alcoholics Anonymous

www.aa.org

Type of Site	Privacy Policy	Advertisements	Direct Sales
Nonprofit	No	No	No

About: Alcoholics Anonymous World Service is a nonprofit, volunteer-based organization headquartered in New York City. According to information found on the Web site, Alcoholics Anonymous's "primary purpose is to stay sober and help other alcoholics to achieve sobriety."

Content: Alcoholics Anonymous presents information about the Alcoholics Anonymous organization (AA), its methods, and its programs. This site also includes general information about alcoholism.

Special Features: Major sections of **Alcoholics Anonymous** include questions and answers about alcoholism and AA, questions and answers for teenagers, and the newsletter *AA Grapevine: 'Our Meeting in Print.'* **Alcoholics Anonymous** is available in English, Spanish, and French.

All Allergy

http://allallergy.net/

Type of Site	Privacy Policy	Advertisements	Direct Sales
Nonprofit	No	Yes	No

About: The CEO, editor, and designer of **All Allergy** is Dr. Harris Steinman, a South African allergist. **All Allergy** is supported by advertisements but does not endorse any products.

Content: All Allergy is a comprehensive allergy resource with links to thousands of allergy-related Web sites. **All Allergy** does not link selectively, but instead aims for comprehensive coverage of allergy information on the Web.

Special Features: Coded symbols indicate the intended audiences of linked Web sites, provide information about the Web site's owner (professional organization, commercial organization, professional's personal site, layperson's site, layperson organization), and rate the Web site's content. A "Daily News" feature provides current information on allergy-related news, and consumers can join the **All Allergy** "Discussion Board."

allHealth.com

www.allhealth.com

Type of Site	Privacy Policy	Advertisements	Direct Sales
Commercial	Yes	Yes	No

About: The **allHealth.com** Web site is the health channel of **iVillage.com: The Women's Network**. In addition to generating revenue through advertisements, **allHealth.com** allows its health topic areas to be sponsored by commercial interests. For example, **allHealth.com**'s section on birth control is sponsored by Ortho-McNeil, a manufacturer of birth control pills.

   Content: Provides original content on many health topics, with the bulk of the information provided covering women's health. Much of this Web site's original content takes the form of questions and answers, with the answers provided by **allHealth.com**'s own medical experts, most of whom are MDs.

   Special Features: Reflecting the **iVillage.com** approach, **allHealth.com** Web site is particularly rich in bulletin boards, chats, support groups, and clubs. Consumers can also subscribe to free **allHealth.com** newsletters covering many diseases and conditions.

Alzheimer's Association

www.alz.org

Type of Site	Privacy Policy	Advertisements	Direct Sales
Nonprofit	No	No	No

About: The largest private funder of Alzheimer's research, the Alzheimer's Association provides education and support for Alzheimer's victims, their families, and their caregivers.

   Content: Besides providing information about the Alzheimer's Association itself, the **Alzheimer's Association** Web site includes sections that provide original content for "People with Alzheimer's," "Family, Caregivers, & Friends," "Physicians & Health Care Professionals," "Researchers," and "Media."

   Special Features: **Alzheimer's Association** provides a glossary of frequently used terms associated with Alzheimer's as well as links to local Alzheimer's Association chapters.

American Academy of Child and Adolescent Psychiatry

www.aacap.org

Type of Site	Privacy Policy	Advertisements	Direct Sales
Nonprofit	Yes	No	Publications

About: The American Academy of Child and Adolescent Psychiatry (AACAP) is a nonprofit association composed of 6,500 child and adolescent psychiatrists and other physicians. AACAP's mission is the "promotion of mentally healthy children, adolescents and families through research, training, advocacy, prevention, comprehensive diagnosis and treatment, peer support and collaboration."

Content: Through its "Facts for Families" section, **American Academy of Child and Adolescent Psychiatry** provides healthcare consumers with nearly 100 original publications dealing with topics ranging from "Making Daycare a Good Experience" to "Teen Suicide." Official translations of "Facts for Families" are available in Spanish; unofficial translations are available in French and German.

Special Features: Additional **American Academy of Child and Adolescent Psychiatry** consumer health resources include "Questions and Answers about Child and Adolescent Psychiatry" and "Glossary of Symptoms and Mental Illnesses Affecting Teenagers."

American Academy of Dermatology

www.aad.org

Type of Site	Privacy Policy	Advertisements	Direct Sales
Nonprofit	No	No	No

About: The American Academy of Dermatology is a membership organization comprised of 13,000 dermatologists in the United States and Canada.

Content: The bulk of the consumer health information found on the **American Academy of Dermatology** Web site comes in the form of patient pamphlets found in the "Patient Education Products" section. There are pamphlets covering specific skin diseases (such as "Acne," "Psoriasis," and "Warts") as well as more general topics (such as "The Darker Side on Tanning," "Mature Skin," and "Poison Ivy, Sumac & Oak"). A few pamphlets are also available in Spanish.

Special Features: A "Find a Dermatologist" feature locates member dermatologists by state. A "Kids' Connection" section provides children from 8 to 18 with information about dermatology and skin health.

American Academy of Pediatrics

www.aap.org

Type of Site	Privacy Policy	Advertisements	Direct Sales
Nonprofit	Yes	No	Publications

About: This is the official Web site of the American Academy of Pediatrics (AAP), a 55,000-member association of pediatricians and pediatric specialists. The mission of AAP "is to attain optimal physical, mental, and social health and well-being for all infants, children, adolescents, and young adults."

Content: The American Academy of Pediatrics "You and Your Family" section provides child and adolescent consumer health information through, among other resources, its "Public Education Brochures" and "The Pediatric Internet" (a list of pediatric Web sites reviewed by pediatricians). The Web site also allows consumers to purchase American Academy of Pediatrics consumer health books directly from AAP.

Special Features: "Media Matters," the national media education campaign of the American Academy of Pediatrics, provides parents with information on how media impacts matters of child and adolescent health.

American Association of Poison Control Centers

www.aapcc.org

Type of Site	Privacy Policy	Advertisements	Direct Sales
Nonprofit	No	No	No

About: The American Association of Poison Control Centers is a nationwide organization of poison centers and interested individuals.

Content: The "Poisoning Prevention and Education" section of the Web site provides poison-related consumer health information, including a printable "Poison Prevention Brochure," "Poison Prevention Fact Sheets," and "Prevention Tips." There is also a "Links" section which leads to other poison resources on the Web.

Special Features: The "Find Your Poison Center" feature allows consumers to search for their local poison control center by interactive map or ZIP code, or by browsing an alphabetical list of poison centers.

American Cancer Society

www.cancer.org

Type of Site	Privacy Policy	Advertisements	Direct Sales
Nonprofit	Yes	No	No

About: The American Cancer Society is the largest source of private, non-profit cancer research funds in the United States. Headquartered in Atlanta, Georgia, the American Cancer Society has over 3,400 local chapters.

Content: American Cancer Society is the Web's leading source for cancer information. The Web site's "Cancer Resource Center" provides consumers with general information about cancer (such as "Prevention & Risk Factors," "Detection & Symptoms," "Types of Treatment") as well as information on specific forms of cancer. Information is available in both English and Spanish.

Special Features: There are substantial sections on "Complementary & Alternative Methods [of Treating Cancer]" and "Living with Cancer."

American Council of the Blind

www.acb.org

Type of Site	Privacy Policy	Advertisements	Direct Sales
Nonprofit	No	No	No

About: The American Council of the Blind (ACB) is the largest U.S. organization for blind and visually impaired people. ACB has 71 affiliated state, regional, and special-interest professional organizations.

Content: The **American Council of the Blind**'s "Helpful Resources" section provides information on such topics as "Catalogs of Products for People Who Are Blind or Visually Impaired," "Guide Dog Schools and Associations," and "Medical Information Sources on Macular Degeneration."

Special Features: Visitors can listen to live Web broadcasts of "ACB Radio." **American Council of the Blind** also offers a collection of articles on pedestrian safety.

American Council on Science and Health

www.acsh.org

Type of Site	Privacy Policy	Advertisements	Direct Sales
Nonprofit	No	No	No

About: The American Council on Science Health (ACSH) is an independent, nonprofit, consumer-education organization. The stated purpose of the ACSH is "to separate the leading causes of disease and death from the leading causes of unnecessary anxiety and . . . to ensure that both individual health decisions and public policies are based on sound scientific evidence."

Content: Sections of the **American Council on Science and Health** Web site cover such topics as "Diseases," "Environmental Health," "Food Safety," and "Medical Care." A main thrust of this Web site is debunking what ACSH sees as alarmist, unscientific stories concerning environmental and technological threats to human health.

Special Features: The "Medical Care" section contains press releases, editorials, and articles that challenge some claims made for alternative therapies. ACSH position papers undergo a peer-review process as described in the "About ACSH" section.

American Diabetes Association

www.diabetes.org

Type of Site	Privacy Policy	Advertisements	Direct Sales
Nonprofit	No	Yes	Publications

About: The American Diabetes Association (ADA) is a nonprofit organization that conducts diabetes programs in all 50 states and the District of Columbia. The association is active in the areas of diabetes research, information, and advocacy. The mission of the American Diabetes Association is to "prevent and cure diabetes and to improve the lives of all people affected by diabetes."

Content: The Web's richest source of consumer health information on diabetes, the **American Diabetes Association** Web site offers sections covering such diabetes-related topics as exercise, nutrition, clinical practice, and more. A "Virtual Grocery Store Tour" (sponsored by food manufacturers) teaches consumers about shopping for a diabetic.

Special Features: Selected articles from the association's consumer magazine *Diabetes Forecast* are available via the Web site. The "Local Info" feature allows consumers to find their nearest ADA office by ZIP code.

American Dietetic Association

www.eatright.org

Type of Site	Privacy Policy	Advertisements	Direct Sales
Nonprofit	Yes	Yes	Publications

About: The American Dietetic Association (ADA) is a professional organization comprised of nearly 70,000 members, the majority of whom are registered dieticians. ADA is the parent organization of the National Center for Nutrition and Dietetics, "an easily accessible, objective source of scientifically-based food and nutrition information."

Contents: Information for healthcare consumers is provided via the "Healthy Lifestyle" and "Knowledge Center" sections of **American Dietetic Association**. Information resources include "Daily Nutrition Tips," "Nutrition Fact Sheets," and a "Good Nutrition Reading List."

Special Features: The "Find a Dietician" feature allows consumers to search for a dietician by ZIP code. Excerpts from the books *Dieting for Dummies* and *The American Dietetic Association's Complete Food & Nutrition Guide* are accessible on this Web site.

American Gastroenterological Association

www.gastro.org

Type of Site	Privacy Policy	Advertisements	Direct Sales
Nonprofit	No	No	No

About: The American Gastroenterological Association (AGA) is a professional association comprised of over 11,000 clinicians, researchers, and educators in the field of gastroenterology.

Contents: The "Public Section" of **American Gastroenterological Association** provides consumer health information, some of it in the form of "AGA Patient Wellness Brochures" covering such topics as "Colorectal Cancer Screening," "Irritable Bowel Syndrome," and "What is Colonoscopy?" A section called "Digestive Health Message Boards" allows consumers to ask and respond to health questions, while the "Gastroenterological Locator Service" allows consumers to find gastroenterologists in their area.

Special Features: Selected full-text articles from *Digestive Health & Nutrition*, a consumer health magazine published by the American Gastroenterological Association, are available via the Web site.

American Heart Association

www.americanheart.org

Type of Site	Privacy Policy	Advertisements	Direct Sales
Nonprofit	Yes	No	No

About: The American Heart Association (AHA) is a privately funded, voluntary health organization with some four million volunteers, and chapters throughout the United States. AHA's stated mission "is to reduce disability and death from cardiovascular diseases and stroke. These include heart attack, stroke (brain attack) and related disorders." Although there are no direct sales on the AHA Web site, there is a link to an online auction from which a percentage of the proceeds go to the AHA.

    Contents: A leading Web site in the areas of heart disease and stroke, **American Heart Association** provides a wealth of consumer health information through its encyclopedic "Heart and Stroke A-Z Guide." Additional information is provided via sections covering "Warning Signs," "Family Health," and "Risk Awareness."

    Special Features: The "Risk Assessment" feature allows consumers to assess their risk for heart attack or stroke via an online quiz. Consumers can enroll in "One Of A Kind," a personalized online health management program.

American Lung Association

www.lungusa.org

Type of Site	Privacy Policy	Advertisements	Direct Sales
Nonprofit	Yes	No	Yes

About: The American Lung Association was founded in 1904 to fight tuberculosis. Today the association and its affiliates around the United States are focused on such health issues as asthma, tobacco control, air pollution, and basic research on lung diseases.

    Content: Besides major sections devoted to "Asthma," "Tobacco Control," and "Air Quality," **American Lung Association** includes a "Diseases A to Z" section that provides information on over 100 lung diseases. A "Links" section points consumers to additional lung-related resources on the Web.

    Special Features: Selected articles from *Asthma Magazine* are available via this Web site. Much information found on **American Lung Association** is available in Spanish as well as English.

American Medical Association

www.ama-assn.org

Type of Site	Privacy Policy	Advertisements	Direct Sales
Nonprofit	Yes	No	No

About: The American Medical Association is the largest physician-member organization in the United States. The association's mission is to be "the nation's leader in promoting professionalism in medicine and setting standards for medical education, practice, and ethics." Though this Web site does sell products directly to physicians, there are no direct sales from the "Patients" section of the site.

Contents: American Medical Association has a "Patients" section, but to a large extent the association provides consumer health information via the **Medem** Web site (see the separate entry later in this chapter).

Special Features: Three features of **American Medical Association** that are of special interest to healthcare consumers are "Doctor Finder," "Hospital Finder," and "Medical Group Practice Finder." All are excellent resources for consumers who wish to identify or obtain information about healthcare providers.

American Podiatric Medical Association

www.apma.org/

Type of Site	Privacy Policy	Advertisements	Direct Sales
Nonprofit	No	No	No

About: The American Podiatric Medical Association (APMA) is the largest association of its kind in the United States, representing approximately 80 percent of all doctors of podiatry in the country. In addition to presenting consumer health information on its Web site, the APMA also provides information via its toll-free number: (800) 366–8227.

Content: The **American Podiatric Medical Association** "Foot Health Information" section provides information on over 40 topics related to foot health, including general and sports-related conditions. The "e-Newsroom" links users to APMA press releases as well as to foot-related full-text articles from newspapers, magazines, and other sources.

Special Features: The "Find a Podiatrist" feature locates doctors of podiatry by ZIP code, while a "Self-Assessment Quiz" allows consumers to answer the question "How Fit Are Your Feet?"

American Psychological Association

www.apa.org/

Type of Site	Privacy Policy	Advertisements	Direct Sales
Nonprofit	Yes	No	Yes

About: With nearly 160,000 members, the American Psychological Association (APA) is the largest psychologist member organization in the world. APA's mission is "to advance psychology as a science, a profession, and a means of promoting human welfare."

Contents: The "Public" section of the **American Psychological Association** Web site provides consumer health information within ten broad areas of interest, including "Mind, Body, & Health," "Minorities," "Parenting & Family," and "Women." Sections titled "News" and "Press Releases" provide information on current topics and controversies from the world of psychology.

Special Features: For consumers, the most useful part of the **American Psychological Association** Web site is the "Help Center" section. It provides access to full-text APA brochures and offers information on such topics as coping with problems at work, using the mind/body connection for better health, dealing with family and relationship problems, and detecting the warning signs of violence. "Help Center" also features the brochure "dotCOMsense," which teaches consumers about such important online issues as guarding one's privacy and evaluating information found on the Net.

AmericasDoctor

http://americasdoctor.com

Type of Site	Privacy Policy	Advertisements	Direct Sales
Commercial	Yes	No	Yes

About: AmericasDoctor is a marketing and pharmaceutical services company sponsored by health organizations in the United States and Canada. The stated purpose of this Web site is to bring together medical researchers, healthcare consumers, hospitals, and Internet resources "to assist the pharmaceutical industry in developing, positioning and promoting its products."

Content: Like so many commercial consumer health Web sites, **AmericasDoctor** provides consumer health information in the form of news reports, a library of short health-related articles, a drug encyclopedia, a medical dictionary, health communities, live Web events, and an "Ask the Doctor" feature.

Special Features: AmericasDoctor provides general information about the nature of clinical trials and allows consumers to register for clinical trials. In addition to its general privacy policy, **AmericasDoctor** has a separate "Clinical Trials Privacy Policy" for those who choose to register to be considered for a clinical trial.

Arthritis Foundation

www.arthritis.org/

Type of Site	Privacy Policy	Advertisements	Direct Sales
Nonprofit	Yes	No	Yes

About: The Arthritis Foundation is a national, voluntary health organization with over 150 chapters and service points in the United States. The Arthritis Foundation's mission "is to support research to find the cure for and prevention of arthritis and to improve the quality of life for those affected by arthritis."

Content: The "Starting Points" and "Arthritis Answers" sections of **Arthritis Foundation** answer common questions about arthritis and provide information on such topics as medications, alternative and complementary therapies, arthritis in children, and the specifics of the more than 100 forms of arthritis.

Special Features: Consumers can read selected articles from the foundation's magazine *Arthritis Today*. A "Message Boards" section allows consumers to exchange information on arthritis-related topics.

ASHA: American Social Health Association

www.ashastd.org/

Type of Site	Privacy Policy	Advertisements	Direct Sales
Nonprofit	Yes	No	No

About: Founded in 1914, the American Social Health Association (ASHA) has the mission "to stop sexually transmitted diseases and their harmful consequences to individuals, families and communities." To this end, ASHA is involved in public awareness, patient education and support, legislative advocacy, and training of healthcare providers.

Content: The consumer health content of **ASHA: American Social Health Association** is found in the Web site's "Facts & Answers about STDS" section. Here consumers will find detailed information on over a dozen major sexually transmitted diseases.

Special Features: An "STD Glossary" defines dozens of medical and scientific terms related to STDs, and a "How to Use a Condom" section provides information on using both male and female condoms and also presents a list of condom do's and don'ts.

Autism Society of America

www.autism-society.org

Type of Site	Privacy Policy	Advertisements	Direct Sales
Nonprofit	No	No	No

About: The Autism Society of America (ASA) was founded in 1965 and now has 18,000 members and over 220 chapters in the United States. According to its own literature, "ASA is dedicated to increasing public awareness about autism and the day-to-day issues faced by individuals with autism, their families and the professionals with whom they interact. The Society and its chapters share a common mission of providing information and education, supporting research and advocating for programs and services for the autism population."

Content: The "Info/Resources" section of **Autism Society of America** offers 20-some information packages under the following headings: "Understanding The Diagnosis," "Education," "Treatment Options," and "Adults With Autism." Some of this information is available in Spanish. Though the quality of the consumer health information on this Web site is high, the amount provided is not large and all of it is in **.pdf** format, which requires the Adobe Acrobat Reader.

Special Features: A "Treatment Comparison Chart" provides consumers with an honest assessment of the advantages and disadvantages of treatments for autism.

Best Doctors

www.bestdoctors.com

Type of Site	Privacy Policy	Advertisements	Direct Sales
Commercial	Yes	No	Yes

About: Best Doctors is a fee-based service intended to help healthcare consumers locate the best doctors by medical specialty and location. According to its own promotional materials, **Best Doctors** is "completely independent. Doctors are not asked for and do not ever pay any fees for inclusion as a Best Doctor."

Content: The heart of **Best Doctors** are its two "Find a Doctor" features. "Best DocFinder" costs $25 and involves an Internet search. "AccuMatch" costs $975 and involves nurses who work with a patient or a patient's representative to locate the best doctor for that particular patient. **Best Doctors** conducts nationwide surveys of doctors to find out which doctors are most recommended by their peers. Only board-certified doctors are included in **Best Doctors,** and doctors who have been sanctioned by state medical boards are excluded.

Special Features: A "Health Information" section provides condition summaries written by medical experts. There is no fee to use the "Health Information" section of **Best Doctors.**

Best Hospitals Finder

www.usnews.com/usnews/nycu/health/hosptl/tophosp.htm

Type of Site	Privacy Policy	Advertisements	Direct Sales
Commercial	Yes	Yes	No

About: **Best Hospitals Finder** is a service of **U.S. News Online,** the Web site of the news magazine *U.S. News & World Report.* The "Rankings" section of **Best Hospitals Finder** explains the methodology used to rank the hospitals selected as the best in the United States.

Content: The bulk of this site is devoted to providing information about top U.S. hospitals. **Best Hospitals Finder** also includes the text of "Best Hospital Articles" from *U.S. News & World Report* as well as links to information on various medical topics.

Special Features: Consumers can choose to see hospitals ranked by specialty and/or geographic region. There is an alphabetical list of all hospitals ranked among the best, as well as a "Best Hospital's Honor Roll."

The Breast Clinic

www.thebreastclinic.com

Type of Site	Privacy Policy	Advertisements	Direct Sales
Nonprofit	No	No	No

About: Based in Glasgow, Scotland, **The Breast Clinic** reflects the efforts of Dr. Stephen Kettlewell (MB, ChB, FRCS), "a surgeon with a specialist interest in breast disease and breast cancer."

Contents: This easy-to-navigate Web site is divided into three sections ("General Information," "Breast Disease," and "Visitor Features") which together provide a complete picture of breast diseases and their treatments.

Special Features: "Discussion Forums" allow consumers to ask and respond to questions relating to breast health and disease. Consumers will find the "Links" section useful for identifying other quality sources of information on breast diseases.

California Poison Control System

www.calpoison.org

Type of Site	Privacy Policy	Advertisements	Direct Sales
Nonprofit	No	No	Yes

About: Administered by the University of California San Francisco, School of Pharmacy, the California Poison Control System (CPCS) is a consortium of California poison control centers. In addition to providing poison hotlines for California, the mission of CPCS is to "educate the public and the health professional community about the prevention and treatment of poisoning."

Content: The "General Public" section of **California Poison Control System** provides a wealth of information on first aid for poisoning, poisonous plants and animals, and how to prevent poisoning. Basic poisoning emergency information is available in 12 languages. The hotline numbers found on this Web site are valid in California only.

Special Features: This Web site includes a "Babysitter's Guide to Poison Prevention," the full text of the *California Poison Control System Answer Book* (in .pdf format), and a nationwide poison control center locator.

Canadian Health Network

www.canadian-health-network.ca

Type of Site	Privacy Policy	Advertisements	Direct Sales
Government	Yes	No	No

About: Founded and funded by Health Canada/Santé Canada, the Canadian Health Network (CHN) provides access to reliable health information from over 600 Canadian organizations.

Content: Canadian Health Network features 26 "Health Centres" covering such major health topics and populations as "Environmental Health," "Aboriginal Peoples," and "Children." The Web site includes over 6,000 links to Internet resources, a 200-question FAQ, and an A–Z index with over 1,000 terms.

Features: The entire Web site is bilingual (English and French). Consumers can access the full text of the *Health! Canada* magazine via **Canadian Health Network**.

CareThere.com

http://carethere.com

Type of Site	Privacy Policy	Advertisements	Direct Sales
Commercial	Yes	No	Yes

About: CareThere.com is a commercial Web site targeted at family caregivers, especially adult children who care for elderly parents. A scientific advisory board and an editorial board, both comprised of medical professionals, provide guidance in regard to the content of **CareThere.com**. Visitors to the Web site can buy health-related products directly from the "CareThere Mall."

Content: Through its "Health Center" and "Library" sections, **CareThere** provides information on health conditions, medications, insurance, and legal matters of interest to family caregivers. The "Communication" section allows consumers to participate in caregiver-centered chats and message boards.

Special Features: Consumers can enter the names of medications they are taking in the site's "Safe Check" feature. "Safe Check" then produces alerts concerning possible drug-drug interactions, drug-food interactions, drug-laboratory interactions, duplicative ingredients, or overlapping drug classes.

Center for Science in the Public Interest

www.cspinet.org

Type of Site	Privacy Policy	Advertisements	Direct Sales
Nonprofit	No	No	No

About: Founded in 1971 the Center for Science in the Public Interest (CSPI) has sought to educate the public and lawmakers in the areas of food safety and nutrition. CSPI publishes the nationally distributed *Nutrition Action Newsletter*. Among other stands, CSPI is strongly opposed to the fat substitute Olestra, genetically modified foods, and alcoholic beverages.

Contents: The focus of **Center for Science in the Public Interest** is food safety and nutrition. To this end the Web site offers "Nutrition Quizzes," reports on food safety and additives, and "News Updates" that often criticize mainstays of the American diet.

Special Features: Consumers can read *Nutrition Action Newsletter* and its monthly "Right Stuff/Food Porn" feature, which employs a witty style to compare healthy foods to high-fat, high-calorie foods.

Centers for Disease Control and Prevention

www.cdc.gov/

Type of Site	Privacy Policy	Advertisements	Direct Sales
Government	Yes	No	No

Contents: Although much Centers for Disease Control and Prevention (CDC) information is aimed at healthcare professionals, a great deal of information at **Centers for Disease Control** can still be of use to consumers. The "Health Topics A–Z" section provides detailed information on hundreds of disease and public health topics. These range from the expected ("Asthma," "E. coli," "Ringworm") to the unexpected ("Cruise Ships," "Ice Hockey," "Tornado"). The "Publications" section includes a number of brochures and guides that could benefit and inform healthcare consumers. Many CDC materials are available in Spanish as well as English.

Special Features: Those who want to go beyond the standard consumer health resources can access the full texts of *MMWR: Morbidity and Mortality Weekly Report* and *Journal of Emerging and Infectious Diseases* via **Centers for Disease Control and Prevention**. The "Travelers' Health" section is probably the best resource of its kind on the Web, and the "Hoaxes and Rumors" section provides a much-needed counter to the various health scares spread via e-mail.

ClinicalTrials.gov

www.clinicaltrials.gov

Type of Site	Privacy Policy	Advertisements	Direct Sales
Government	Yes	No	No

About: Developed by the National Library of Medicine, **ClinicalTrials.gov** is a service of the National Institutes of Health.

Contents: ClinicalTrials.gov provides information about thousands of clinical studies; most of these studies are sponsored by federal agencies, but there are plans to add studies sponsored by the pharmaceutical industry as well. Consumers can search for clinical trials by keyword or browse by either condition or sponsor. Once a study is found, **ClinicalTrials.gov** provides information on the study's purpose, its eligibility requirements, location, and contact information.

Special Features: The "Resources" section of **ClinicalTrials.gov** provides consumers with information that explains what is involved in a clinical trial and why someone might, or might not, wish to volunteer for one.

Discoveryhealth.com

http://health.discovery.com

Type of Site	Privacy Policy	Advertisements	Direct Sales
Commercial	Yes	Yes	Yes

About: Discoveryhealth.com is an offshoot of the Discovery Health Channel, a commercial television channel that delivers programming relating to health, medicine, and wellness.

Contents: Within the "Disease and Conditions" section of **Discoveryhealth.com**, four online encyclopedias (*Diseases & Conditions, Injuries, Surgery,* and *Medical Tests*) provide substantial, signed articles on hundreds of health-related topics; in most cases, the authors of these articles are medical doctors.

Special Features: The "Health Tools" section features "Calculators," "Assessments," and "Trackers" that allow consumers to assess and monitor their own health.

DoctorDirectory.com

www.doctordirectory.com

Type of Site	Privacy Policy	Advertisements	Direct Sales
Commercial	No	Yes	Yes

About: A privately owned company based in Asheville, North Carolina, **DoctorDirectory.com** provides direct-to-consumer and direct-to-physician interactive marketing services to the healthcare industry.

Contents: DoctorDirectory.com is the flagship of a related group of Web sites, including **HospitalDirectory.com, ClinicalTrialDirectory.com, MedicalSchoolDirectory.com, HealthPlanDirectory.com,** and **HealthNews Directory.com.** The titles of **DoctorDirectory.com** and its sister Web sites give a good indication of the kind of information each site provides. For example, consumers can use **DoctorDirectory.com** to search for doctors by specialty or name/location, use **HospitalDirectory.com** to look up U.S. hospitals by location, and use **HealthPlanDirectory.com** to get information about health plans around the country. **HealthNewsDirectory.com** connects consumers to current health information supplied by many of the Web's leading news outlets.

Special Features: The "Sanction Search" feature allows consumers to see if a particular doctor has been sanctioned. For a fee, consumers can order a license/sanction report that spells out the disciplinary action taken against the sanctioned physician.

drkoop.com

www.drkoop.com

Type of Site	Privacy Policy	Advertisements	Direct Sales
Commercial	Yes	Yes	Yes

About: Headed by former U.S. Surgeon General C. Everett Koop, **drkoop.com** is a commercial Web site that "strives to be the most trusted and complete source of consumer healthcare information and services on the Internet." In addition to providing consumer health information, **drkoop.com** develops Web-based health tools and enters into partnerships with commercial affiliates. Launched with much fanfare in 1999, **drkoop.com** has struggled financially.

Contents: Sections such as "Family Health," "Health & Wellness," and "Conditions & Concerns" provide access to original consumer health information, message boards, health tools (such as "Asthma Calculator" and "Ideal Weight Calculator"), and links to health resources that have been rated by **drkoop.com**'s own experts.

Special Features: Visitors to **drkoop.com** can view health-related videos on such topics as menopause, teen safety, stroke recovery, and more.

eMD

www.emd.com

Type of Site	Privacy Policy	Advertisements	Direct Sales
Commercial	Yes	No	Yes

About: The Internet healthcare company eMD is a subsidiary of BioShield Technologies, based in Norcross, Georgia. The mission of eMD "is to offer a comprehensive solution that decreases healthcare costs—while improving the quality of patient care by reducing medication errors, increasing compliance, and improving outcomes."

Content: The eMD Web site consists of both a physician site and a consumer site. The consumer site's "Health Conditions" section provides substantial information on 1,700 individual health topics. As with many commercial consumer health sites, consumers can e-mail health-related questions to healthcare professionals retained by the Web site. According to **eMD**, consumers who send questions can "expect a response within one (1) business day."

Special Features: The "Healthy Home" and "Healthy Habits" sections provide preventive measures consumers can take to maintain good health.

Epilepsy Foundation

www.efa.org

Type of Site	Privacy Policy	Advertisements	Direct Sales
Nonprofit	Yes	No	Publications

About: The Epilepsy Foundation is a national nonprofit organization with over 60 affiliates nationwide. The mission of the Epilepsy Foundation is "to work for children and adults affected by seizures through research, education, advocacy and service."

Content: An extremely well-organized and easy-to-navigate Web site, **Epilepsy Foundation** presents the bulk of its consumer health information via its "Answer Place" section. Within the "Answer Place," consumer health information is accessible by topic (such as "Treatment," "Medications," and "First Aid") or by audience (such as "Adults," "Parents," and "Police/Law Enforcement"). Additional consumer health information can be found in the "Epilepsy USA News" and "Services" sections.

Special Features: The "e-Communities" section allows consumers to interact with others who have similar epilepsy-related interests.

extendedcare.com

http://extendedcare.com

Type of Site	Privacy Policy	Advertisements	Direct Sales
Commercial	Yes	No	No

About: The **extendedcare.com** Web site is a service of Extended Care Information Network, an Internet company that connects "hospitals and consumers with extended-care providers, including nursing homes, assisted-living and other senior-living residences, and home health care agencies." In addition to providing information on senior health issues, Extended Care Information Network produces business software products for hospitals and extended care facilities.

Content: The consumer health content of **extendedcare.com** is found under the site's "For Everyone" link. The "Informed Living" section provides signed articles (most written by social workers or other healthcare professionals) on such care-related topics as "Healthy Sexuality," "Financial Planning," "Pharmacy Facts," and "Health Maturity." The "Library" section provides access to chapters (most written by MDs or PhDs) with such titles as "Influenza Vaccine Update," "High Blood Pressure," and "Drug Interactions."

Special Features: A sophisticated "Provider Finder" allows consumers to search for care facilities by location and/or name. In addition, a search can be narrowed by such factors as language criteria, method of payment, and size of facility. Over 70,000 U.S. care providers are included in the "Provider Finder" database.

Family Doctor

www.familydoctor.co.nz

Type of Site	Privacy Policy	Advertisements	Direct Sales
Nonprofit	Yes	No	No

About: Based in New Zealand, **Family Doctor** is funded by private individuals and overseen by an editorial board comprised of medical professionals.

Content: Consumer health information is what **Family Doctor** is all about, and the database-driven nature of this Web site makes it easy to find pertinent information, whether you search by one of the broad categories (such as "Women's Health" or "Sports Health") or one of the "A to Z Conditions." All the consumer health information provided by **Family Doctor** is signed, dated, and written in an easy-to-understand, nonintimidating style.

Special Features: Not only can consumers register for the **Family Doctor** e-mail newsletter, but they can customize it by indicating what health topics are of special interest. Registration for the newsletter requires only an e-mail address.

familydoctor.org

www.familydoctor.org

Type of Site	Privacy Policy	Advertisements	Direct Sales
Nonprofit	No	No	No

About: The **familydoctor.org** Web site is a service of the American Academy of Family Physicians, a national association of family doctors with over 93,000 members in the United States. Founded in 1947, the academy's purpose is "to promote and maintain high quality standards for family doctors who are providing continuing comprehensive health care to the public." According to a statement found on **familydoctor.org**, "All of the information within **familydoctor.org** has been written and reviewed by physicians and patient education professionals at the American Academy of Family Physicians. The information is regularly reviewed and updated."

Content: An especially bountiful source of consumer health information, **familydoctor.org** provides consumers with numerous "Health Info Handouts," "AAFP Family Health Facts," and flowcharts for "Self-Care." (The latter are decision trees that help patients decide what steps to take based on symptoms and other factors.) Many of the "Health Info Handouts" are available in Spanish as well as English.

Special Features: The **familydoctor.org** Web site provides plentiful information (taken from Micromedex) on "Herbal and Alternative Remedies."

FirstGov

www.firstgov.gov

Type of Site	Privacy Policy	Advertisements	Direct Sales
Government	Yes	No	No

About: A service of the U.S. government, **FirstGov** is "the first-ever government Web site to provide the public with easy, one-stop access to all online U.S. Federal Government resources."

Content: The "Healthy People" section of **FirstGov** provides access to U.S. government information on health (via **healthfinder** [*www.healthfinder.gov*]), insurance, and disease (via **National Institutes of Health: Health Information** [www.nih.gov/health]).

Special Features: The **FirstGov** keyword search allows consumers to pull up information from every U.S. government Web resource.

Food and Drug Administration

www.fda.gov

Type of Site	Privacy Policy	Advertisements	Direct Sales
Government	Yes	No	No

About: The U.S. Food and Drug Administration (FDA) is the federal agency charged with regulating food, medical devices, drugs, biologicals (such as vaccines and blood products), animal feed and drugs, cosmetics, and radiation-emitting consumer and medical products. FDA is under the U.S. Department of Health and Human Services.

Content: For the areas over which FDA has regulatory control, **Food and Drug Administration** provides access to extensive consumer health information. Most of this information can be accessed via the site's "Consumer," "Patients," "Women," "Seniors," and "Kids" sections. Visitors to the site can also access the full text of *FDA Consumer*, a magazine published by FDA.

Special Features: The "Buying Medicines and Medical Products Online" feature helps consumers be more informed and cautious when doing their online shopping.

Galaxy

http://galaxy.einet.net

Type of Site	Privacy Policy	Advertisements	Direct Sales
Commercial	Yes	Yes	No

About: Founded in 1994 **Galaxy** is a for-profit Web directory owned by a subsidiary of Fox Entertainment and a group of private investors. Galaxy accepts advertisements and sponsorships of its "Vertical Targeted Directories."

Content: Similar to **Yahoo!** in that it covers a full range of subject areas, **Galaxy** provides links to consumer health information via its "Medicine" section (though within this section there is no division between consumer and professional information). Once in the "Medicine" section, consumers can click down through the directory structure until they find a link to the information they need. There is no original health information on **Galaxy**.

Special Features: Instead of relying entirely on retrieval technology, **Galaxy** employs degreed librarians to compile and organize its Web site so that the information it provides will be contextually relevant and have high content value.

Go Ask Alice!

www.goaskalice.columbia.edu

Type of Site	Privacy Policy	Advertisements	Direct Sales
Educational	Yes	No	Publications

About: Go Ask Alice! is a service of Alice!, Columbia University's Health Education Program, itself a division of the Columbia University Health Service.

Content: Using a question-and-answer format, **Go Ask Alice!** strives to provide factual, nonjudgmental information about physical, sexual, emotional, and spiritual health. **Go Ask Alice!** has generated controversy by providing frank answers to questions about sex posted by children and teens.

Special Features: The **Search Alice!** feature allows consumers to search an archive of 1,800 previously answered questions. **Go Ask Alice!** allows consumers to post questions anonymously.

Health Care Financing Administration

www.hcfa.gov

Type of Site	Privacy Policy	Advertisements	Direct Sales
Government	Yes	No	No

About: The Health Care Financing Administration is the U.S. government agency responsible for administering Medicare, Medicaid, and the State Children's Health Insurance Program.

Content: The "Information for Beneficiaries" link is the most direct way to access the consumer information contained on **Health Care Financing Administration**. Besides providing information on such topics as "Medicare Private Fee-for-Service Plans" and "Maternal AIDS Consumer Information," **Health Care Financing Administration** makes numerous links to its companion Web sites **Medicare** (*www.medicare.gov*) and **Insure Kids Now** (*www.insure kidsnow.gov*).

Special Features: Although the companion Web sites listed above have more information on their specific topics, **Health Care Financing Administration** makes a good starting point because it ties together all the major federal health insurance programs.

Health on the Net Foundation (HON)

www.hon.ch

Type of Site	Privacy Policy	Advertisements	Direct Sales
Nonprofit	Yes	No	No

About: Founded in 1995 the **Health on the Net Foundation (HON)** is a Swiss nonprofit organization whose mission "is to guide the growing community of healthcare consumers and providers on the World Wide Web to sound, reliable medical information and expertise." Major sponsors of HON a. Microsystems, the Swiss Institute of Bioinformatics, and the State of Geneva.

Content: A gateway to health information, **HON** features MedHunt (an intelligent search engine designed to locate Web-based health information) and HONselect (a database of quality health information on the Web).

Special Features: The HON Code of Conduct (HON Code) is a set of eight principles intended to promote quality and honesty in the provision of health information via the Web. Sites that feature the HON Code logo have agreed to uphold these principles.

HealthAnswers

www.healthanswers.com/

Type of Site	Privacy Policy	Advertisements	Direct Sales
Commercial	Yes	Yes	No

About: HealthAnwers, based in Austin, Texas, is a for-profit company that provides consumer health information in conjunction with *Physicians Weekly*, Reuters Health Information, Gold Standard Multimedia, and other content partners.

Content: In the nascent genre of for-profit consumer health Web sites, **HealthAnswers** is a classic of the type. Via the site's "Health Centers," "Health Topics," or "Diseases/Conditions" sections, consumers can find large amounts of original consumer health information on thousands of topics. The site also features a drug database in both English and Spanish, a collection of some 2,000 audio/video segments on various health topics, health chat rooms, and current health news. Any visitor who completes a free registration can set up a customized "My Health" page.

Special Features: A "Visual Search Tool" allows consumers to find information on disease and conditions by pointing and clicking on a human figure.

healthAtoZ.com

http://healthatoz.com

Type of Site	Privacy Policy	Advertisements	Direct Sales
Commercial	Yes	Yes	No

About: Medical Network is the parent company of both the consumer-oriented **healthAtoZ** and a sister Web site for healthcare professionals,

MedConnect.com (also known as **healthAtoZProfessional**). Founded by an MD, **healthAtoZ** is overseen by a medical advisory board composed of medical doctors and pharmacists. Although there are now no direct sales on **healthAtoZ**, information on the site reports that "online transactions" will soon be available.

Content: Within sections titled "Your Family," "Condition Forums," "Wellness Centers," and "Healthy Lifestyles," **healthAtoZ** provides both original content and links to rated and reviewed Web sites. Other features include "my healthatoz," health-related message boards, online chats with health experts, and assorted calculators (such as weight, fertility, and fitness).

Special Features: Consumers who complete a free registration can use **healthAtoZ**'s "eMate," a Web-based software application which, among other things, functions as an online health record organizer, allows users to keep online food and exercise journals, and sends e-mail reminders about checkups, prescription refills, and immunizations.

HealthCentral

www.healthcentral.com

Type of Site	Privacy Policy	Advertisements	Direct Sales
Commercial	Yes	Yes	Yes

About: California-based **HealthCentral** is a for-profit health Web site that generates profits through advertising and direct sales of health-related products. **HealthCentral**'s chief medical officer, an MD, is responsible for "medical content and quality related issues" on the Web site.

Content: A typical large, for-profit health Web site, **HealthCentral** provides access to consumer health information via a "Conditions & Topics" section as well as through "Topic Centers" and a searchable "Library and Encyclopedias" section. There are also sections that offer health calculators, access to support communities, drug information, and information on alternative health topics. At times the lines between consumer health information and product sales are blurred on this Web site.

Special Features: Consumers can subscribe to 50 health-related newsletters. The site offers regular features by celebrity doctor Dean Edell.

healthfinder

www.healthfinder.gov

Type of Site	Privacy Policy	Advertisements	Direct Sales
Government	Yes	No	No

About: A service of the U.S. Department of Health and Human Services, **healthfinder** is "a gateway to selected consumer health and human services information resources provided by U.S. government agencies and other organizations serving the public interest."

Content: As a gateway Web site, **healthfinder** provides links to resources rather than providing original information. The bulk of the linked resources are U.S. government Web sites. Every linked resource must meet the criteria of the **healthfinder** selection policy, which consumers may read on the **healthfinder** site. Consumers can find information on a wide variety of health topics by using the **healthfinder** search engine, by using the site's alphabetical index, or by exploring various categories. A good deal of health information in Spanish is accessible via **healthfinder**.

Special Features: By clicking the "details" link provided for each linked resource, consumers can learn about the resource before choosing whether or not to visit it. A new companion site, **healthfinder Kids**, provides links to age-appropriate information for those under 18.

HealthGrades

www.healthgrades.com

Type of Site	Privacy Policy	Advertisements	Direct Sales
Commercial	Yes	Yes	No

About: HealthGrades "educates and empowers consumers by offering free objective ratings and in-depth profiles that allow them to evaluate and select providers based on quality." In addition to selling advertisements, **HealthGrades** syndicates its content to other Web sites and sells custom ratings and directories to employers and healthcare plans.

Content: The heart of **HealthGrades** is its "Healthcare Report Cards" which rate hospitals, physicians, nursing homes, home health agencies, hospice programs, and fertility clinics. Consumers can search for report cards in a number of ways, including by name, state, ZIP code, medical specialty, and so on. The site also includes a "Conditions A–Z" section.

Special Features: In its "Grading Methodologies" section, **HealthGrades** provides detailed descriptions of how it determines its ratings and what these ratings mean.

HealthHelper.com

http://healthhelper.com

Type of Site	Privacy Policy	Advertisements	Direct Sales
Commercial	Yes	No	Yes

About: California-based **HealthHelper.com** provides health information both to consumers and healthcare professionals The medical director of **HealthHelper.com** is Joe Jacobs, MD, MBA, the original director of the National Institutes of Health Office of Alternative Medicine.

Content: The main divisions of **HealthHelper.com** are "Complementary Health," "Conventional Health," "Health4Youth," and "Vitamins and Supplements." This site is particularly strong in presenting information on complementary (alternative) medicine, and the information it provides is generally well balanced. The "Ask Nurse Nancy" feature allows consumers to post medical questions to a registered nurse, and the "Health4Youth" section presents health information aimed at younger children, teens, and parents.

Special Features: A "Drug Interactions" feature (which is somewhat buried in the "Botanical Medicines" section of "Complementary Health") provides valuable information on drugs, herbs, and nutrients.

HealthWeb

www.healthweb.com

Type of Site	Privacy Policy	Advertisements	Direct Sales
Government	No	No	No

About: A project of the health sciences libraries of the Greater Midwest Region (GMR) of the National Network of Libraries of Medicine (NN/LM) and of the Committee for Institutional Cooperation, **HealthWeb** organizes and provides access to evaluated, noncommercial, health-related, Internet-accessible resources.

Content: A gateway site, **HealthWeb** primarily provides links to Web resources rather than providing original information. The simple, easy-to-navigate **HealthWeb** homepage lists 60-some categories of health information.

The links found under these categories point to sites aimed at healthcare professionals as well as sites for healthcare consumers.

Special Features: The **HealthWeb** "User Guides" help consumers make effective use of such Web resources as MEDLINE and document-delivery services. They also give guidance on how to evaluate Web resources and on how to search the Web.

HealthWorld Online

www.healthy.net

Type of Site	Privacy Policy	Advertisements	Direct Sales
Commercial	No	Yes	Yes

About: California-based **HealthWorld Online** promotes what it calls "Self-Managed Care,"™ an approach that strives for a synthesis of alternative and conventional health care. The **HealthWorld Online** board of directors includes both conventional and alternative practitioners.

Content: Organized around the concept of a small town, **HealthWorld Online** is divided into such areas as "Fitness Center," "University," "Marketplace," and "Alternative Medicine." Though there is some inclusion of conventional medicine, **HealthWorld Online** clearly favors alternative health care and provides large doses of information on alternative health therapies, medicines, diets, lifestyles, and providers.

Special Features: The **HealthWorld Online** "Medical Cybrarian" service provides consumers with customized medical research for a fee of $50 per hour.

HIV InSite

http://hivinsite.ucsf.edu

Type of Site	Privacy Policy	Advertisements	Direct Sales
Educational	No	No	No

About: A service of the University of California San Francisco (UCSF) Positive Health Program at San Francisco General Hospital Medical Center and of the UCSF Center for AIDS Prevention Studies (both of which are programs of the UCSF AIDS Research Institute), **HIV InSite** is supported by sponsors that range from Merck to the National Institute of Mental Health to the San Francisco Giants baseball team. According to the **HIV InSite** editorial policy, "**HIV InSite**

strives to provide a fair and balanced representation of viewpoints on many controversial aspects of AIDS." Supporters of **HIV InSite** have no say in editorial decisions, which are based on the "credibility, reliability, and accuracy" of the information in question.

Content: One of the richest sources of HIV and AIDS information on the Web, **HIV InSite** is divided into sections that cover, among other things, the clinical, social, and prevention aspects of the disease. One section of the site is entirely devoted to Spanish-language information resources.

Special Features: The "Audio Archives" section of **HIV InSite** allows consumers to access audio and audio/video presentations of HIV/AIDS information.

InteliHealth

www.intelihealth.com

Type of Site	Privacy Policy	Advertisements	Direct Sales
Commercial	Yes	Yes	Yes

About: Billing itself as "The Trusted Source®," **InteliHealth** strives to provide reliable consumer health information from sources that include Harvard Medical School and the University of Pennsylvania School of Dental Medicine. **InteliHealth** is owned and partly funded by Aetna U.S. Healthcare.

Content: Consumers can access consumer health information under such categories as "Men's Health," "Women's Health," "Children's Health," and "Senior's Health," or they can search by condition. **InteliHealth** offers health-related chat, a "Drug Resource Center," an "Ask the Doc" feature, health news, and free health e-mails on nearly 20 topics.

Special Features: Because of its partnership with the University of Pennsylvania School of Dental Medicine, **InteliHealth** is a particularly good source for information on oral health.

KidsHealth

www.kidshealth.com

Type of Site	Privacy Policy	Advertisements	Direct Sales
Nonprofit	Yes	No	No

About: A service of the Nemours Foundation Center for Children's Health Media, the mission of **KidsHealth** "is to provide the best children's health information on the Internet." A large team of health professionals serve as medical reviewers for **KidsHealth**. The Nemours Foundation also operates the Alfred I. duPont Hospital for Children and several Nemours Children's Clinics in Florida.

Content: The **KidsHealth** Web site is divided into three main sections ("Parents," "Kids," and "Teens") each of which contains consumer health information appropriate for its target audience. Each of these divisions provides a large amount of original content on a wide variety of topics, such as "Bringing Your Baby Home" (Parents), "Migraines: What a Pain" (Kids), and "Toxic Shock Syndrome" (Teens).

Special Features: The "Game Closet" features a number of online games (such as "Health Hunt" and "How the Body Works") that allow kids to learn about health while having fun.

MayoClinic.com

www.mayoclinic.com

Type of Site	Privacy Policy	Advertisements	Direct Sales
Nonprofit	Yes	No	No

About: Owned by the Mayo Foundation for Medical Education and Research through its subsidiary HealthOasis, **MayoClinic.com** "is produced by a team of writers, editors, multimedia and graphics producers, health educators, nurses, doctors, and scientists." All information on the site is developed and/or reviewed by Mayo Clinic health professionals and is based on scientific research. Formerly, **MayoClinic.com** was known as **Mayo HealthOasis**.

Content: Consumers may access original consumer health information via "Diseases and Conditions," "Condition Centers," or "Healthy Living Centers." **MayoClinic.com** allows consumers to search for information on over 8,000 prescription and over-the-counter medications via its "Drug Information" feature, while a "First-Aid & Self-Care Guide" covers dozens of major and minor health problems.

Special Features: All information on **MayoClinic.com** is dated and reviewed annually to ensure that it remains current and accurate.

Medem

www.medem.com

Type of Site	Privacy Policy	Advertisements	Direct Sales
Commercial	Yes	No	No

About: A joint venture among eight of the leading medical societies in the United States, **Medem** "provides innovative tools and secure technologies for physicians to provide patients access to trusted health information via their doctor's own Web site."

Content: The heart of **Medem** is its "Medical Library." Divided into four sections ("Life Stages," "Diseases and Conditions," "Therapies and Health Strategies," and "Health and Society") the "Medical Library" consist of peer-reviewed information provided by medical societies.

Special Features: The "Physician Finder" feature allows consumers to search for a physician via "AMA Physician Select," or "Find an EyeMD," or "The ACOG [American College of Obstetricians and Gynecologists] Physician Directory," or "The ASPS Plastic Surgeon Referral Service."

MEDLINE*plus*

www.medlineplus.gov

Type of Site	Privacy Policy	Advertisements	Direct Sales
Government	Yes	No	No

About: A service of the U.S. National Library of Medicine, **MEDLINE*plus*** primarily organizes and provides links to full-text consumer health publications of the National Institutes of Health and other U.S. federal government organizations. **MEDLINE*plus*** also links to nongovernment Web sites that meet its criteria for quality and accessibility.

Content: MEDLINE*plus* is composed of five major divisions: "Health Topics," "Drug Information," "Dictionaries," "Directories," and "Other Resources." The links in the "Health Topics" section number in the hundreds. Most health topics include links to significant numbers of Spanish-language publications.

Special Features: Visitors to MEDLINE*plus* have free access to the *ADAM Medical Encyclopedia*.

Medscape

www.medscape.com

Type of Site	Privacy Policy	Advertisements	Direct Sales
Commercial	Yes	No	No

About: Medscape is a provider of digital health records and online health information. **Medscape**'s mission is "to improve healthcare by delivering products and services that provide reliable, digital clinical data and up-to-date information to healthcare professionals and consumers." The editor in chief of **Medscape** is George Lundberg, MD, former editor of *JAMA: The Journal of the American Medical Association.*

Content: Although **Medscape** is aimed more at healthcare professionals than at consumers, it contains a wealth of health information for the diligent consumer. **Medscape** offers a large and searchable collection of free, full-text medical articles as well as consumer-oriented information. To access much of **Medscape**, visitors must complete a free registration process.

Special Features: Its partnership with **CBS HealthWatch** makes **Medscape** one of the best places on the Web for accessing current health news.

Merck Manual of Medical Information—Home Edition

www.merck.com/pubs/mmanual_home/contents.htm

Type of Site	Privacy Policy	Advertisements	Direct Sales
Commercial	No	No	No

About: Merck is an international biomedical company involved in publishing and the development and manufacture of pharmaceuticals.

Content: Based on *The Merck Manual of Diagnosis and Therapy* (aka *The Merck Manual*), the **Merck Manual of Medical Information—Home Edition** is very much in the tradition of the one-volume encyclopedia of home health. The 287 chapters and 5 appendixes of the **Merck Manual of Medical Information—Home Edition** provide a wealth of scientifically based health information for the consumer. Chapters range from "Pain" to "Nutritional Disorders" to "Cataracts."

Special Features: The high caliber of the editors, consultants, contributors, and the editorial/production staff make the **Merck Manual of Medical Information—Home Edition** one of the most trustworthy consumer health resources on the Web.

National Women's Health Information Center

www.4woman.gov

Type of Site	Privacy Policy	Advertisements	Direct Sales
Government	Yes	No	No

About: A service of the U.S. Department of Health and Human Services Office on Women's Health, **National Women's Health Information Center** (NWHIC) links to U.S. federal government as well as other women's health information resources. The mission of NWHIC "is to provide current, reliable, commercial and cost-free, health information to women and their families."

Content: The bulk of the consumer health information found on **National Women's Health Information Center** can be accessed via the extensive alphabetical listings found under "Health Topics" or via keyword search. The **National Women's Health Information Center** homepage provides current news on women's health issues as well as such topic links as "Men's Health," "Body Image," and "Violence Against Women."

Special Features: As with **HealthFinder**, clicking the "Details" link provided for each Web resource listed on **National Women's Health Information Center** brings up descriptive information about the resource.

NetWellness

www.netwellness.org

Type of Site	Privacy Policy	Advertisements	Direct Sales
Nonprofit	Yes	No	No

About: A nonprofit, consumer health resource, **NetWellness** "provides high quality information created and evaluated by medical and health professional faculty at the University of Cincinnati, Case Western Reserve University, and The Ohio State University." The original content found on **NetWellness**, as well as the linked Web sites, must "meet the Health Summit Working Group Criteria for credibility, content and disclosure."

Content: The alphabetical links in the **NetWellness** "Health Topics" section lead to signed and dated original content, evaluated links, or topic-specific "Ask an Expert" pages. Other sections of **NetWellness** include "Today's News," "Library," and "Clincial Trials."

Special Features: The "TeenLook@Health" section of **NetWellness** provides teenagers with health information created by a partnership of medical school faculty, medical students, and high school technology students.

NOAH: New York Online Access to Health

www.noah-health.org

Type of Site	Privacy Policy	Advertisements	Direct Sales
Nonprofit	No	No	No

About: NOAH: New York Online Access to Health is a service of the City University of New York, the Metropolitan New York Library Council, the New York Academy of Medicine, and the New York Public Library. Currently funded by Federal Library Services and Technology Act funds granted by the New York State Library, **NOAH** also receives support from the Queens Borough Public Library, the March of Dimes, Aetna U.S. Healthcare, and NYU Medical Center. "**NOAH** seeks to provide high quality full-text health information for consumers that is accurate, timely, relevant and unbiased. **NOAH** currently supports English and Spanish."

Content: A gateway Web site, **NOAH** provides links to consumer health information via its "Health Topics" section.

Special Features: NOAH is one of the best gateways on the Web for locating consumer health information in Spanish.

NORD

www.rarediseases.org

Type of Site	Privacy Policy	Advertisements	Direct Sales
Nonprofit	Yes	No	Yes

About: The National Organization for Rare Disorders (NORD) is composed of 140 "voluntary health organizations dedicated to helping people with rare 'orphan' diseases and assisting the organizations that serve them." According to **NORD**, a rare disease is any disease that "affects fewer than 200,000 people in the United States." Although visitors to **NORD** can purchase products intended for those who suffer from rare diseases, there is a clear division between the nonprofit part of **NORD** and its "Marketplace" section.

Content: The heart of **NORD** is its three databases. The "Rare Disease Database" provides consumer-oriented information on over 1,000 rare diseases. The "Organizational Database" helps consumers get in touch with associations, foundations, agencies, and support groups that assist those affected by rare diseases. The "Orphan Drug" database provides information on some 900 drugs that have been designated as Orphan Drugs by the U.S. Food and Drug Administration.

Special Features: NORD is distinguished by the fact that it provides consumer health information that is otherwise difficult or impossible to find—even for those who have access to the Web and know how to search it.

OncoLink

www.oncolink.org

Type of Site	Privacy Policy	Advertisements	Direct Sales
Nonprofit	Yes	Yes	No

About: Founded in 1994 **OncoLink** is a service of the University of Pennsylvania Cancer Center. The mission of **OncoLink** is "to help cancer patients, families, health care professionals and the general public get accurate cancer-related information at no charge." **OncoLink** is funded in part by a number of corporate sponsors, most of which are pharmaceutical manufacturers.

Content: A rich and easy-to-navigate source of cancer information aimed at both healthcare consumers and professionals, **OncoLink** is divided into such sections as "Disease Oriented Menus," "Cancer Causes, Screening, and Prevention," "Clinical Trials," and "Financial Issues for Patients." Much of the information on **OncoLink** is original content, and all such content is signed and dated.

Special Features: "OncoLink TV" uses RealMedia Video to present videos on such topics as specific diseases and supportive care for cancer patients.

pain.com

www.pain.com

Type of Site	Privacy Policy	Advertisements	Direct Sales
Nonprofit	No	Yes	Publications

About: A subsidiary of the Dannemiller Memorial Educational Foundation, **pain.com** is also supported by educational grants from a number of biomedical corporations. According to its detailed "Advertisement Policy," **pain.com** closely controls advertising on its Web site and does not permit the advertising of specific products. Although there is no privacy policy, **pain.com** does subscribe to the HON Code of Conduct of the Health on the Net Foundation.

Content: Divided into "Professional Information" and "Consumer Information" sections, **pain.com** provides links to pain resources on the Web, a directory of pain clinics in the United States and abroad, a searchable "Pain Library," a directory of pain support groups, and an "Ask the Pain Doctor" feature.

Special Features: A "Pain Assessment Tools" feature provides printable scales and surveys that consumers can print out and use to communicate the extent of their pain to their healthcare provider.

Partnership for Caring

www.partnershipforcaring.org

Type of Site	Privacy Policy	Advertisements	Direct Sales
Nonprofit	No	No	Publications

About: The Partnership for Caring: America's Voices for the Dying is a nonprofit organization that brings together individuals, organizations, consumers, and professionals to improve end-of-life care.

Content: The "Resources" section of **Partnership for Caring** offers a variety of end-of-life information resources aimed at consumers, including a "Glossary of Terms" associated with end-of-life issues, articles from *Voices: The Newsletter of the Partnership for Caring*, and a number of useful fact sheets. In the "Advanced Directives" section, consumers can download state-specific packages that help the dying and their families make sure the wishes of the dying are respected to the extent that the laws of the various states permit.

Special Features: The "Family and Consumer Resource Guide" (located in the **Partnership for Caring** "Toolbox" section) contains both original content as well as links to outside resources that help the dying and their families plan and prepare for an impending death.

PDR.net

www.pdr.net

Type of Site	Privacy Policy	Advertisements	Direct Sales
Commercial	Yes	Yes	Publications

About: The online arm of the venerable drug reference book *Physician's Desk Reference*,[1] **PDR.net** is owned by the New Jersey-based Medical Economics Company, a division of Thompson Healthcare.

Content: The "For Consumers" section of **PDR.net** includes sections titled "Drug Information," "PDR for Herbal Medicines," "Health News," and "PDR's Getting Well Network," the latter providing information on about a half-dozen conditions commonly treated with medication. (At least one of the "Getting Well Network" areas is sponsored by the manufacturer of a pharmaceutical used to treat the condition in question.) Users who complete a free registration may access three subsections of "Drug Information": PDR® Family Guide to Prescription Drugs, PDR® Family Guide to Women's Health, and PDR® Family Guide Encyclopedia of Medical Care. A fourth subsection— PDR (Physician's Desk Reference)—is accessible only to consumers who pay a fee of $10 per month or $100 per year.

Special Features: Consumers may access the first edition (1998) of *PDR for Herbal Medicines* free of charge.

PersonalMD.com

www.personalMD.com

Type of Site	Privacy Policy	Advertisements	Direct Sales
Commercial	Yes	Yes	Yes

About: PersonalMD.com is a California-based commercial Web site that generates income through advertising and online retail sales. A medical advisory board composed of nine MDs reviews the content of the site for relevance and accuracy.

Content: Like many other commercial consumer health Web sites, **PersonalMD.com** provides access to information on a number of diseases and conditions. However, the centerpiece of **PersonalMD.com** is its online medi-

---

1. *Physicians' Desk Reference*. Montvale, NJ: Medical Economics Company, Inc., 2001.

cal records feature. For a fee of $40 per year, an individual can store his or her medical records on the secure **PersonalMD.com** Web site. Those who subscribe to this service are issued a card containing information that, in an emergency, allows a physician or other healthcare provider to access the patient's online medical record.

Special Features: Subscribers to the **PersonalMD.com** online medical records service can receive pager reminders to take medication, have access to an online calendar that keeps track of medical appointments—and sends e-mail reminders, and can make use of the "ER-call" feature that notifies emergency contacts if a subscriber is taken to an emergency room.

RealAge

www.realage.com

Type of Site	Privacy Policy	Advertisements	Direct Sales
Commercial	Yes	Yes	Yes

About: **RealAge** bills itself as an "infomediary" that connects consumers with advertisers. Advertisements are sent to **RealAge** members only with the permission of the member and are tailored to conform to the member's stated interests.

Content: The philosophy informing **RealAge** is based on the idea that proper health and lifestyle choices can reduce one's chronological age to a more youthful "real age." To this end, the **RealAge** "Lifestyle Centers," "Health Assessments," and "Home Health" sections present information designed to promote youth and good health. The **RealAge** "Medical Encyclopedia" contains a substantial number of articles on health topics of interest to seniors (and others). Most of these articles are signed, either by MDs or other appropriate health professionals.

Special Features: Those who complete the free registration can sign up to receive *HealthBytes*, a customizable electronic newsletter that includes consumer health information as well as product advertisements.

RxList

www.rxlist.com

Type of Site	Privacy Policy	Advertisements	Direct Sales
Commercial	Yes	Yes	Yes

About: Founded by a pharmacist, **RXList** is now a Healthcentral Network partner.

Content: RxList provides detailed information on thousands of drugs. Consumers can simply type the name of a drug into the **RxList** search box or use the site's "Advanced Search" feature to do fuzzy or keyword searches of all the **RxList** drug monographs (of which there are 4,500 written in "plain English" and 3,000 in "plain Spanish"). Consumers can also search for information on alternative medications such as herbal remedies and homeopathics.

Special Features: The **RxList** "Top 200 Drugs" feature provides links by generic drug name to monographs on the most prescribed medications.

SafetyAlerts.com

www.safetyalerts.com

Type of Site	Privacy Policy	Advertisements	Direct Sales
Commercial	Yes	Yes	No

About: A service of Michigan-based Safe-T-net, **SafetyAlerts.com** was established by Paul M. Walsh to present and distribute "safety related recall information regarding contaminated food and faulty products sold in the United States."

Content: The homepage of **SafetyAlerts.com** presents current news about U.S. product recalls. Consumers can also access information about recalls by category (for example, "Food," "Clothing," and "Toys") or search the Web site for specific information.

Special Features: Consumers can sign up for e-mail safety alerts that can be customized to include only those alerts that impact the user's state and/or only certain categories or brands of products.

Shape Up America!

www.shapeup.org

Type of Site	Privacy Policy	Advertisements	Direct Sales
Nonprofit	No	No	Yes

About: Founded by former U.S. Surgeon General C. Everett Koop, **Shape Up America!** is the product of a coalition of nonprofit organizations concerned with improving health in the United States. **Shape Up America!** is wholly financed by the private funds of corporations, commodity boards, and foundations. The mission of **Shape Up America!** is "to educate the public on the importance of the achievement and maintenance of a healthy body weight through the adoption of increased physical activity and healthy eating."

Content: Emphasizing a scientific approach to weight management that emphasizes health eating and physical activity, **Shape Up America!** provides consumers with such features as a "CYBERkitchen" (which helps them develop a customized, balanced diet and provides healthy recipes), a "Body Fat Lab" (which explains what body fat is and allows consumers to calculate their own body fat), and a "Fitness Center" (which helps consumers create a sensible exercise plan).

Special Features: For a fee of $10 per week, consumers can join the "Shape Up & Drop 10" diet and exercise program.

*the*health*channel*.com

www.thehealthchannel.com

Type of Site	Privacy Policy	Advertisements	Direct Sales
Commercial	Yes	Yes	Yes

About: California-based *the*health*channel*.com is a commercial Web site that generates income through advertising, direct sales (to both healthcare consumers and professionals), and business-to-business services.

Content: Billing itself as a "Total Health Care Web site offering quality content and interactive health care management products for both the consumer and professional markets," *the*health*channel*.com offers the usual array of consumer health information, online health communities, and online services (such as "Personal Health Record" and "Body Mass Index Calculator").

Special Features: The "Symptoms & Conditions Finder" (which is found in the "Reference Tools Section") allows consumers to select one or more symptoms from a list of several hundred symptoms and retrieve relevant original articles as well as relevant information from **MEDLINE***plus*.

thriveonline

http://thriveonline.oxygen.com

Type of Site	Privacy Policy	Advertisements	Direct Sales
Commercial	Yes	Yes	Yes

About: A service of the media company Oxygen (parent of cable channel **oxygenTV**), **thriveonline** is a commercial Web site that generates income through advertising and online retail sales.

Content: One of the most heavily visited consumer health sites on the Web, **thriveonline** follows the usual practice of large, commercial consumer health Web sites by offering information via such features as a disease and conditions section, health centers, and a medical library. This site also supports health communities, an ask-an-expert feature, and personal health calculators.

Special Features: The focus of **thriveonline** is women's health.

Virtual Hospital

www.vh.org

Type of Site	Privacy Policy	Advertisements	Direct Sales
Nonprofit	No	No	No

About: **Virtual Hospital** is a service of the University of Iowa Health Care, a partnership between the University of Iowa College of Medicine and University of Iowa Hospitals and Clinics.

Content: One of the richest and best organized sources of consumer health information on the Web, **Virtual Hospital** provides information to consumers via its "For Patients" and "Common Problems" sections. Consumers can browse by department or organ system to find relevant articles from the *Iowa Health Book*. All these articles are signed, include a date of creation and date of last review, and provide information on their peer-review status. **Virtual Hospital** also offers **Virtual Children's Hospital**, a Web site that provides consumer health information for both parents and children.

Special Features: **Virtual Hospital** is an especially good resource for anyone who wants to learn about a specific medical procedure, including why a procedure is performed, how it is performed, and what is involved in recovery.

WebMD

www.webmd.com

Type of Site	Privacy Policy	Advertisements	Direct Sales
Commercial	Yes	Yes	Yes

About: A commercial health Web site, **WebMD** provides health news and information for both healthcare consumers and professionals. A five member health advisory board (four MDs and a PhD) oversees the content on the site, and **WebMD** posts explicit policy statements regarding content, advertising, and the editorial independence of its "WebMD National News Center."

Content: The "Consumer Health" section of **WebMD** offers all the services expected on a large, commercial consumer health Web site: a disease and conditions section, health centers, health communities, an ask-an-expert feature, personal health calculators, and online medical records.

Special Features: As perhaps the most frequently visited, heavily advertised, and well-financed consumer health site on the Web, **WebMD** provides more information and services than the average Web site.

Yahoo! Health

http://dir.yahoo.com/Health

Type of Site	Privacy Policy	Advertisements	Direct Sales
Commercial	Yes	Yes	Yes

About: **Yahoo! Health** is part of the **Yahoo!** directory, perhaps the oldest, best known, and most heavily used directory on the Web. Yahoo! is a commercial company that generates income via advertising and online sales to consumers. Web sites listed on **Yahoo!** can pay to be featured more prominently than they normally would be.

Content: A gateway Web site, **Yahoo! Health** may have more links to health-related Web sites than any other site on the Internet. Users can access content via the **Yahoo!** directory structure or by using the **Yahoo!** search engine.

Special Features: The downside of **Yahoo! Health** is that Web sites are listed regardless of the quality of their content; thus links to quack Web sites may be listed right alongside links to the most reliable and accurate health information on the Web.

5

Recommended Consumer Health Print Resources

There is no shortage of print resources on consumer health information. In recent years, books have appeared on every subject from common diseases and symptoms to complementary and alternative health care. The vast number of titles that could be added to a consumer health collection makes it difficult for a librarian with a limited budget to decide which titles to buy. Suggestions on how to select books for a particular collection include:

- Purchase books on topics that reflect health concerns of your geographic area. For example, air quality is a major concern in Houston, Texas, so books on respiratory disease are essential for a consumer health collection in Houston.
- Purchase books from a reputable health or scientific vendor.
- Select books that are written by well-known experts in the fields (for example, a book by Dr. Michael DeBakey on heart disease) or published by a major health institution (such as the Mayo Clinic or Johns Hopkins University).
- Consult well-known medical book lists, especially those by Brandon/Hill, published in the *Bulletin of the Medical Library Association*.
- Since currency is important in medicine, only purchase books published within the last three years unless a title is a known "classic" in the field.
- Sometimes you can identify a really good health series—such as the Omnigraphics *Health Reference Series* (some titles from this series are listed below)—that can help fill major gaps in a collection.
- Contact a local hospital or academic medical center library to see what core reference books they recommend.
- Partner with a local hospital or academic medical center library for referrals and interlibrary loans of materials not available.
- Work with local medical librarians or the regional National Network of Libraries of Medicine[1] to provide your library staff with classes on medical information.

---

1. The mission of the National Network of Libraries of Medicine (NN/LM) is to "advance the progress of medicine and improve the public health by: 1) providing all U.S. health professionals with equal access to biomedical information; and, 2) improving the public's

In this chapter the authors provide some examples of titles, in specific health areas, that are appropriate for a small or medium-sized consumer health collection. This is in no way meant to be an exhaustive list, only a starting point for collection development staff members.

Acquired Immune Deficiency Syndrome (AIDS)

Bartlett, John G., and Ann K. Finkbeiner. *The Guide to Living with HIV Infection*. Baltimore: Johns Hopkins University Press, 1998.
> Developed by the Johns Hopkins AIDS Clinic, this book includes medical issues, psychological and social issues, and questions and answers about HIV infection. The book covers the parts of people's lives that HIV infection affects including physical health, emotional health, social difficulties, and financial and legal problems. The book is written by health professionals, but an opening disclaimer stresses that the book is not meant to be a substitute for medical care; rather it was written to improve communication between the patient and the health professional.

Bellenir, Karen, ed. *AIDS Sourcebook*. Detroit: Omnigraphics, 1999.
> Offers information on both AIDS and HIV, including updated statistical data, reports on recent research and prevention initiatives, new antiretrovial treatment options, strategies for combating opportunistic infections, and information about clinical trials. Also included are a glossary and a list of additional resources.

Frumkin, Lyn R., and John M. Leonard. *Questions and Answers on AIDS*. Los Angeles: Health Information Press, 1997.
> Written by two physicians and in its third edition, this collection concerns the myriad issues surrounding the HIV/AIDS epidemic and is addressed to both the caregivers and those infected by the HIV virus. Issues addressed include the cause, transmission, diagnosis, epidemiology, manifestations, and treatment of HIV/AIDS; opportunistic infections; and HIV and public policy.

Kaiser, Jon D. *Healing HIV: How to Rebuild Your Immune System*. Mill Valley, Calif.: HealthFirst Press, 1998.
> This book, written by a physician, contains over 20 case histories, including some concerning difficult-to-treat patients. The author compares pa-

access to information to enable them to make informed decisions about their health. The Program is coordinated by the National Library of Medicine and carried out through a nationwide network of health science libraries and information centers." To contact the NN/LM office nearest you call (800) 338–7657.

tients who received conventional HIV treatment with those whose treatment included major herbs from both Western and Chinese medical traditions. These latter patients were treated in consultation with herbalists experienced with HIV.

Alzheimer's Disease

Bellenir, Karen, ed. *Alzheimer's Disease Sourcebook*. Detroit: Omnigraphics, 1999.

Offers information on Alzheimer's disease and related disorders, including multi-infarct dementia, AIDS-related dementia, alcoholic dementia, Huntington's disease, delirium, and confusional states. Also included are reports of current research efforts in prevention and treatment, long-term care issues, and a list of additional resources.

Ewing, Wayne. *Tears in God's Bottle: Reflections on Alzheimers Caregiving*. Tucson, Ariz.: Whitestone Circle Press, 1999.

A personal account by the author, this is the story of Wayne Ewing and his wife of 40 years, Ann Margaret Wentz Ewing. When Ann was diagnosed with Alzheimer's, Wayne took on the role of a caregiver. Illustrating the pain and frustration, along with the enormous responsibility, this book helps to share experiences with others who might be affected by this relentless disease. The book is both an important revelation for those who share the tragedy of Alzheimer's as well as a deeply moving testament of love and the human spirit of caring for others.

Kuhn, Daniel. *Alzheimer's Early Stages: First Steps in Caring and Treatment*. Alameda, Calif.: Hunter House, 1999.

A product of the Rush Alzheimer's Disease Center in Chicago, this book focuses on the medical aspects of Alzheimer's disease, including a normal aging pattern of the brain and the effects of the disease. Also discussed are long-term planning, relationships, communication, and staying healthy while caring for someone with Alzheimer's.

Mace, Nancy L., and Peter V. Rabins. *The 36-Hour Day: A Family Guide to Caring for Persons with Alzheimer Disease, Related Dementing Illnesses, and Memory Loss in Later Life*. Baltimore: Johns Hopkins University Press, 1999.

In its third edition, this book was especially written for families and friends of those suffering from Alzheimer's disease, dementia, and memory loss. The authors include new information on laws, financing and delivery of care, assisted living, eating and nutrition, medical research on drugs, genetics, and diagnostic tests.

Roche, Lyn. *Coping with Caring: Daily Reflection for Alzheimer's Caregivers.* Forest Knolls, Calif.: Elder Books, 1996.

>A wonderful resource written for those who care for a loved one with Alzheimer's or a related disorder. With great emphasis on the wellbeing of the caregiver, the author provides an inspiring daily reflection followed by related caregiving tips. Designed for daily use, this book includes a handy 10-page index for quick reference to over 200 challenges caregivers might encounter, including wandering, sundowning, caregiver stress, and anger.

Cancer

Dollinger, Malin, Ernest H. Rosenbaum, and Greg Cable. *Everyone's Guide to Cancer Therapy: How Cancer Is Diagnosed, Treated, and Managed Day to Day.* Kansas City, Mo.: Andrews McMeel, 1997.

>In this third edition of *Everyone's Guide to Cancer Therapy,* the authors present a comprehensive guide to dealing with cancer, including diagnosis, treatment, and supportive care. This edition updates all the information from previous editions including new treatment methods, new discoveries, and new research directions. The book also includes plentiful illustrations and diagrams, a thorough listing of cancer associations and support groups, and a glossary.

Finn, Robert. *Cancer Clinical Trials: Experimental Treatments and How They Can Help You.* Sebastopol, Calif.: O'Reilly, 1999.

>This book, intended for anyone who has been diagnosed with cancer as well as caregivers of those with cancer, offers advice on treatment options and clinical trials. The author discusses reasons for deciding in favor of or against participating in a trial; the structure, administration, and ethical guidelines of clinical trials; who is included and excluded from joining clinical trials; how to read the informed consent document and trial protocol; and includes a set of hard questions patients must ask themselves and their doctors.

Fromer, Margot Joan. *Surviving Childhood Cancer: A Guide for Families.* See the section "Children" later in this chapter.

Janes-Hodder, Honna, and Nancy Keene. *Childhood Cancer: A Parent's Guide to Solid Tumor Cancers.* See the section "Children" later in this chapter.

Johnston, Lorraine. *Colon and Rectal Cancer: A Comprehensive Guide for Patients and Families.* Sebastopol, Calif.: O'Reilly, 2000.

Offers information on the characteristics of colon cancer, including s
ing, suspected causes, and factors in prognoses; current treatment oৄ
tions; clinical trials; coping with medical tests, symptoms, and treatments;
minimizing the impact on sexuality and fertility; emotional responses to
diagnosis, treatment, and remission; and caring for and adjusting to an
ostomy.

Keene, Nancy. *Childhood Leukemia: A Guide for Families, Friends, and Caregivers*. 2d ed. Beijing: O'Reilly, 1999.

Childhood leukemia is the most common of all childhood cancers, each
year afflicting some 2,500 children in the United States. Written by a
mother whose own daughter was diagnosed with the disease, *Childhood
Leukemia* takes a sequential approach to its subject, beginning with a
chapter on diagnosis and moving on to cover such medical topics as hospitalization, chemotherapy, radiation, and working with healthcare providers. In addition, the author addresses such emotional and social aspects of the disease as its impact on family and friends, school, behavior,
and more. Readers will find the chapter on record-keeping and finances
especially helpful.

Keene, Nancy, Wendy Hobbie, and Kathy Ruccione. *Childhood Cancer Survivors: A Practical Guide to Your Future*. See the section "Children" later in this chapter.

Levin, Bernard. *Colorectal Cancer: A Thorough and Compassionate Resource for Patients and Their Families*. New York: Villard, 1999.

Published under the auspices of the American Cancer Society, this book
contains some of the most up-to-date information about colon and rectal
cancers, including basic facts about what to do when confronted with a
diagnosis; the latest medical data, treatments and procedures; and recipes
and diet plans to help alleviate stress on the body. The author also offers
psychological and emotional support through case histories to which patients can relate.

Mayer, Musa. *Advanced Breast Cancer: A Guide to Living with Metastatic Disease*. 2d ed. Beijing: O'Reilly, 1998.

This book deals with all aspects of breast cancer, including coping with
the shock of recurrence; making treatment decisions; communicating effectively with medical personnel; managing symptoms of disease progres-
sion; treatment of side effects; getting emotional support from other patients, friends, and family; and finding new ways to keep hope alive and
discover meaning in the midst of adversity.

McKay, Judith, and Ancee Hirano. *The Chemotherapy and Radiation Therapy Survival Guide: Information, Suggestions, and Support to Help You Get Through Treatment*, Oakland, Calif.: New Harbinger Publications, 1998.
>   Since most people facing cancer therapy have no idea of what lies ahead, this book explains what chemotherapy and radiation therapy are, how they work, and how they may affect the patient. The authors also answer common questions and give practical suggestions about what the patient can do to help himself or herself while receiving treatment.

Murphy, Gerald P., Lois B. Morris, and Dianne Lange. *Informed Decisions: The Complete Book of Cancer Diagnosis, Treatment, and Recovery*. New York: Viking, 1997.
>   Written under the auspices of the American Cancer Society, the purpose of this book is to present comprehensive information so that patients diagnosed with one of over 100 diseases classed as cancer can make informed critical choices. The book will help them understand the options available, feel secure in the choice of health care professionals and treatment facilities, comprehend recommendations made by health care professionals, organize and evaluate the vast amounts of information available, be sure the best possible care is provided, remain in control, and alleviate fear and anxiety.

Prucha, Edward J. *Cancer Sourcebook*. Detroit: Omnigraphics, 2000.
>   Offers information about major forms and stages of cancer and features facts about primary and secondary tumors of specific organs as well as tumors of the respiratory, nervous, lymphatic, circulatory, skeletal, and gastrointestinal systems. Coverage includes statistical and demographic data, treatment options, strategies for coping, a glossary, and a directory of additional resources.

Prucha, Edward J., ed. *Pediatric Cancer Sourcebook*. See the section "Children" later in this chapter.

Runowicz, Carolyn D., Jeanne A. Petrek, Ted S. Gansler, and Dianne Lange. *Women and Cancer: A Thorough And Compassionate Resource for Patients and Their Families*. New York: Villard, 1999.

Wilkes, Gail M., and Terri B. Ades. *Consumer's Guide to Cancer Drugs*. See the section "Drugs and Herbals" later in this chapter.

Children

American Medical Association. *Complete Guide to Your Children's Health.* New York: Random House, 1999.

> This encyclopedia of children's most common health problems includes chapters on the various age levels, from newborn to teenager; a complete safety guide on babyproofing and childproofing a home; an atlas of a child's body; a diagnostic skin rash chart; a first-aid and emergency care guide; a growth chart; and more than 20 symptom charts to help determine what is wrong with a sick child.

Complete Directory for Pediatric Disorders. Lakeville, Conn.: Grey House, 2000.

> This book was written with three goals in mind: to meet the growing consumer demand for current, understandable medical information on pediatric disorders, conditions, and diseases; to provide an extensive overview of the educational resources and support services available for parents and children; and to serve as a comprehensive resource for physician assistants, case workers, genetic counselors, librarians, and other professionals who are dedicated to providing concerned parents and other caregivers with vital supportive services.

Fromer, Margot Joan. *Surviving Childhood Cancer: A Guide for Families.* Oakland, Calif.: New Harbinger Publications, 1998.

> This guide is designed to help families cope with the ways that cancer changes the lives of the afflicted child, the parents, siblings, other family members, and friends. The author describes the illness and its treatment, offers advice on how to cope with emotions and stress, discusses how to talk about the illness with the child and others, tells where to find information and help, and explains how to develop honest and trusting relationships with medical caregivers.

Geralis, Elaine, ed. *Children with Cerebral Palsy: A Parents' Guide.* Bethesda, Md.: Woodbine House, 1998.

> Offers comprehensive coverage of the subject of children with cerebral palsy, including diagnosis, assessment, adjustment, therapies, early intervention, special education, legal rights, daily care, family life, development, medical treatment, and advocacy.

Gershwin, M. Eric, and Edwin L. Klingelhofer. *Taking Charge of Your Child's Allergies: The Informed Parent's Comprehensive Guide.* Totowa, N.J.: Humana Press, 1998.

> The authors answer basic questions that parents ask about a child with

allergies. The book is divided into five sections, including a general introduction to childhood allergies; identifying and avoiding triggers of allergy; diagnosis, treatment, and control of allergies; the role allergies play in general health; and strategies to follow to provide an antigen-free environment.

Janes-Hodder, Honna, and Nancy Keene. *Childhood Cancer: A Parent's Guide to Solid Tumor Cancers*. Sebastopol, Calif.: O'Reilly, 1999.
For the 6,000 children in the United States being treated for solid tumor cancers (neuroblastoma, Wilms tumor, liver tumors, bone sarcomas, retinoblastoma), the authors have provided information on the basic understanding of medical terminology, chemotherapy, and common side effects of treatment. They also cover diagnosis to the end of treatment, relapse, and bereavement; practical advice on dealing with procedures, hospitalization, school, family, friends, and financial issues; and how to work effectively with medical personnel.

Keene, Nancy, Wendy Hobbie, and Kathy Ruccione. *Childhood Cancer Survivors: A Practical Guide to Your Future*. Sebastopol, Calif.: O'Reilly, 2000.
More than 250,000 children, teens, and adults in the United States are survivors of childhood cancer. The authors have written a guide that provides these survivors with information on late medical effects from treatment, emotional aspects of surviving cancer, schedules for follow-up care, challenges in the healthcare system, lifestyle changes to maximize health, and discrimination in employment and insurance.

Prucha, Edward J., ed. *Pediatric Cancer Sourcebook*. Detroit: Omnigraphics, 1999.
This book contains information about the cancers that are most often diagnosed in infants, children, and adolescents, including leukemias, brain tumors, sarcomas, lymphomas, and other types of pediatric cancer. The author provides disease descriptions, treatment options, alternative therapies, tips on finding specialized cancer centers and organizations, and a special section on financial assistance and working with health insurance companies. Also included are suggestions for parents, caregivers and concerned relatives, a glossary of cancer terms, and a list of additional resources.

Schwartz, M. William, ed. *The 5 Minute Pediatric Consult*. 2d ed. Philadelphia: Lippincott, Williams & Wilkins, 2000.
This basic reference covers over 1,000 topics arranged alphabetically and cross-indexed to synonyms, including chief complaints, specific diseases,

syndromes, and herbal treatments. There is also a surgical glossary. This second annual edition offers a quick medical reference for current medical diagnosis and treatment.

Swanson, Jennifer. *Infant and Toddler Health Sourcebook*. Detroit: Omnigraphics, 2000.
> Offers information about the physical and mental development of newborns, infants, and toddlers, including neonatal concerns, nutritional recommendations, immunization schedules, common pediatric disorders, assessments and milestones, safety tips, and advice for parents and other caregivers. Also includes a glossary and a resource list.

Complementary and Alternative Medicine

Dillard, James, and Terra Ziporyn. *Alternative Medicine for Dummies*. Foster City, Calif.: IDG Books Worldwide, 1998.
> Defining alternative medicine as any health care practice that is not usually emphasized in conventional medical schools, the authors focus on how to determine when alternatives are worth a try and when they might be dangerous; how to evaluate various alternative approaches; how to use alternative medicine safely; how to find a convenient doctor who is open to alternative treatment; and how to find an alternative practitioner.

Horstman, Judith. *The Arthritis Foundation's Guide to Alternative Therapies*. Atlanta: Longstreet Press, 1999.
> This consumer's guide covers healing systems, mind-body connections, exercise alternatives, massage acupuncture, copper bracelets, magnet therapy, elimination diets, and information on over 40 herbs and supplements.

Hudson, Tori. *Women's Encyclopedia of Natural Medicine: Alternative Therapies and Integrative Medicine*. See the section "Women's Health" later in this chapter.

Marti, James. *Holistic Pregnancy and Childbirth*. New York: John Wiley & Sons, 1999.
> Discusses the latest therapies, techniques, and natural approaches to pregnancy and childbirth. Topics addressed include acupuncture and acupressure, aromatherapy, diet and nutrition, exercise, homeopathy, osteopathy, and yoga.

Murray, Michael, and Joseph Pizzorno. *Encyclopedia of Natural Medicine: Your Comprehensive, User-Friendly A-to-Z Guide to Treating More than 70 Medical Conditions—From Arthritis to Varicose Veins, from Cancer to Heart Disease.* 2d ed. Rocklin, Calif: Prima Health, 1998.

> This completely revised and expanded second edition provides information on the healing powers of natural medicine. Writing in easy-to-read language, yet basing what they write on scientific research, the authors advise readers on the natural approach to treating over 70 diseases.

Rister, Robert. *Japanese Herbal Medicine: The Healing Art of Kampo.* See the section "Drugs and Herbals" later in this chapter.

Williams, Tom. *The Complete Illustrated Guide to Chinese Medicine: A Comprehensive System for Health and Fitness.* Boston: Element Books, 1999.

> Even though Chinese medicine has been around for over 3,000 years, it has never been as popular in the Western world as it is now. This illustrated guide covers the basic principles behind Chinese medicine, the meridian system and how it works, the causes of disharmony, treatments (including acupuncture, herbal remedies, nutrition, qigong, and meditation), and the future of Chinese medicine in Western medicine.

Death

Davies, Phyllis. *Grief: Climb Toward Understanding.* San Luis Obispo, Calif.: Sunnybank, 1998.

> Written after the author's son was killed in an airplane collision, this book includes practical information in dealing with grief. Included are checklists, proactive choices on how to prepare for a death, suggestions on dealing with someone who is seriously ill or dying, and helping children when someone close to them dies. Also discussed are decisions to be made when someone dies, examples of living wills, dealing with the funeral home, communication with family and friends, and creating memorials.

Kolf, June Cerza. *Comfort and Care in a Final Illness: Support for the Patient and Caregiver.* Tucson, Ariz.: Fisher Books, 1999.

> The author, a long-time hospice coordinator and bereavement director, divides her book into two sections, one for the patient and one for the caregiver. Chapters aimed at the patient include information on physical considerations, emotional adjustments, and spiritual approaches. Chapters aimed at the caregiver include information on the role of the caregiver, caring for the patient, final arrangements, and understanding death.

Kolf, June Cerza. *How Can I Help: How to Support Someone Who Is Grieving*. Tucson, Ariz.: Fisher Books, 1999.

> This supportive resource is aimed not at the person who is closest to the deceased, but to other helpers who come in contact with the griever. Written in four parts, the author divides grief support into time segments: the initial contact, the week after the funeral, the first six months, and the one-year anniversary.

Lynne, Joanne, Joan Harrold, and the Center to Improve Care of the Dying. *Handbook for Mortals: Guidance for People Facing Serious Illness*. New York: Oxford University Press, 1999.

> Produced by George Washington University, this handbook provides practical information for people facing serious illness, the death of a loved one, and the decisions that must be made in such situations. With a caring approach, such topics as death of a child, living with serious illness, making decisions, talking with the doctor, controlling pain, and enduring loss are all discussed.

Diabetes

Bellenir, Karen, ed. *Diabetes Sourcebook*. Detroit: Omnigraphics, 1998.

> Offers information on Type 1 and Type 2 diabetes, gestational diabetes, and related disorders, as well as information on prevalence data, management issues, the role of diet and exercise in controlling diabetes, insulin and other medicines, and related complications (such as eye diseases, periodontal diseases, amputation, and end-stage renal disease). Also included are reports on current research initiatives, a glossary, and a list of additional resources.

Keane, Maureen, and Daniella Chace. *What to Eat if You Have Diabetes: A Guide to Adding Nutritional Therapy to Your Treatment Plan*. Lincolnwood, Ill.: Contemporary Books, 1999.

> The goal of this book is to help patients, their families, and caregivers develop meal plans based on fresh whole-plant foods while creating an individualized program for regular blood sugar control. Also included is an easy-to-understand overview of the disease and how food affects someone diagnosed with diabetes.

Levin, Marvin E., and Michael A. Pfeiffer, eds. *The Uncomplicated Guide to Diabetes Complications*. Alexandria, Va.: American Diabetes Association, 1998.

> Using lay language, the authors provide in-depth coverage of diabetes complications, including kidney and heart disease, eye disease and blind-

ness, hypertension and stroke, neuropathy and vascular disease, skin and dental problems, and impotence and sexual disorders. They also discuss such special concerns as obesity and hypoglycemia.

Loring, Gloria. *Parenting a Child with Diabetes*. 2d ed. Chicago, Ill.: Contemporary Books, 2000.

This book is a practical survival guide for parents who have children suffering from diabetes. Written by a parent whose son was diagnosed with the disease in 1979, Ms. Loring provides a manual that teaches other parents everything they need to know about caring for a diabetic child without upsetting delicate family dynamics or destroying the family's physical or emotional well being.

Drugs and Herbals

Bellenir, Karen. *Drug Abuse Sourcebook*. Detroit: Omnigraphics, 2000.

Offers information about illicit substances and the diversion of prescription medications, including depressants, hallucinogens, inhalants, marijuana, narcotics, stimulants, and anabolic steroids. Also includes facts about related health risks, treatment issues, and substance abuse prevention programs; a glossary; statistical data; and directories.

Fetrow, Charles W., and Juan R. Avila. *The Complete Guide to Herbal Medicines*. Springhouse, Pa.: Springhouse, 2000.

Produced by the St. Francis Medical Center in Pittsburgh, this book serves as a guide to over 300 herbal medicines. Coverage includes uses for each herb, recent research, common doses, side effects, interactions, references to scientific studies, and nonherbal alternative medicines.

Foster, Steven, and Varro E. Tyler. *Tyler's Honest Herbal: A Sensible Guide to the Use of Herbs and Related Remedies*. New York: Haworth Herbal Press, 1999.

Provides botanical information as well as folkloric background of herbal remedies. Also included are both positive and negative effects of the most important therapeutic herbs.

Graedon, Joe, and Teresa Graedon. *Dangerous Drug Interactions*. New York: St. Martin's Press, 1999.

Helps the reader understand the dangerous interactions that can occur when mixing medicines, food, and vitamins. The authors offer over 200 easy-to-understand charts with information on medications for pain relief, allergies, asthma, arthritis, heart problems, depression, diabetes, contraception, and ulcers. They also include special information for women, children, and older adults.

Medical Economics. *PDR: Physicians' Desk Reference*. Montvale, N.Y.: Medical Economics, 2001.
> A core drug reference title, the *PDR* is listed as a "core and first-purchase" selection by Brandon/Hill. The *PDR* is an annual compilation of labeling information for FDA-approved prescription drugs and includes photographs of the drugs.

Medical Economics. *The PDR Family Guide to Prescription Drugs*. 6th ed. New York: Random House, 1998.
> The goal of this book is to make the many benefits of modern pharmaceuticals, as well as the risks, as clear and simple as possible. Included are all the important side effects, no matter how rare, attributed to each drug by the manufacturer. Standard dosage recommendations are also included, as are instructions on what to do when a dose is missed or in the case of an overdose. Drugs are listed by their familiar brand names with cross references to generic names.

Rister, Robert. *Japanese Herbal Medicine: The Healing Art of Kampo*. Garden City Park, N.Y.: Avery Publishing Group, 1999.
> Originating in China, Kampo is the herbal system of healing based on observation of symptoms. This book is divided into two parts. The first part is a discussion of what Kampo is, including how to buy and use herbs. In the second part the author discusses how to use to herbs to treat over 100 disorders such as asthma, cancer, and yeast infections.

Rybacki, James J. *Essential Guide to Prescription Drugs*. New York: Harper Perennial, 1998.
> Offers detailed, comprehensive information on the most important drugs in current use, including suggestions for how consumers can lower their prescription costs. Information on specific drugs includes benefits versus the risks of taking the drug, generic and brand names, whether a drug is available generically, principal uses of the drug, how the drug works, possible side effects on sexuality, if a drug is safe to take while pregnant or breastfeeding, and precautions for patients over 60.

Wilkes, Gail M., and Terri B. Ades. *Consumer's Guide to Cancer Drugs*. Sudbury, Mass.: Jones and Bartlett, 2000.
> Produced by the American Cancer Society and the Boston Medical Center, this book answers common drug-related questions in lay language.

Included are lists of the most common drugs on the market today along with the drug's action, how to take the drug, precautions, side effects, and other important facts.

Fertility and Sexuality

Marcaccio, Amy. *Family Planning Sourcebook*. Detroit: Omnigraphics, 2000.
Offers information about planning for pregnancy, contraception (traditional methods, barrier methods, permanent methods, future methods, emergency contraception), and birth control choices for women at each stage of life. Also included are statistics, a glossary, and sources of additional information.

Matthews, Dawn D. *Sexually Transmitted Diseases Sourcebook*. Detroit: Omnigraphics, 2000.
Includes information on the diagnosis and treatment of chlamydia, gonorrhea, hepatitis, herpes, HIVC, mononucleosis, and syphilis. Also includes information on prevention of STDs through condom use, vaccines, and STD education; a section on issues related to youth and adolescents; a glossary; and a list of additional resources.

Peoples, Debby, and Harriett Rovner Ferguson. *What to Expect When You're Experiencing Infertility: How to Cope with the Emotional Crisis and Survive*. New York: W. W. Norton, 1998.
This book is divided into 12 chapters grouped according to the four stages involved in resolving infertility: crisis, acceptance, resolution, and treatment.

Steidle, Christopher P. *The Impotence Sourcebook*. Los Angeles: Contemporary Publishing Group, 1998.
The purpose of this book is to help the reader recognize, prevent, and treat impotence. Includes information on working with a doctor to determine emotional and physiological causes and explore treatment options; drug treatments, including organ medications, injections, and testosterone therapy; maintenance of sexual health; and different types of surgery that might improve erectile functioning.

Turiel, Judith Steinberg. *Beyond Second Opinions: Making Choices About Infertility*. Berkeley, Calif.: University of California Press, 1998.
Discusses the risks, errors, and distortions surrounding fertility medicine and serves as a guide for those seeking treatment. The author uses up-to-date medical literature to shed new light on difficult decisions patients face today on reproductive questions.

Heart Disease, High Blood Pressure, and Stroke

American Medical Association Guide to Hypertension. New York: Pocket Books, 1998.

> Offers clear, concise information on understanding all aspects of hypertension (high blood pressure), how the body controls hypertension, treatable causes, how to safely monitor blood pressure, taking control of health with lifestyle recommendations, and working with your doctor on maintaining a drug therapy program. Also includes information about hypertension and African Americans, children, seniors, pregnant women, and people with diabetes; answers to commonly asked questions; a glossary; and a list of additional resources.

Burkman, Kip. *The Stroke Recovery Book.* Omaha: Addicus Books, 1998.

> The author, a rehabilitation physician, offers advice on how strokes occur, what happens to the brain during strokes, major types of strokes and their effects, cognitive (personality, emotional, intellectual, and behavioral) changes, speech and language impairments, weakness in limbs, swallowing problems, recovery and rehabilitation, and stroke prevention.

Sheps, Sheldon G., ed. *Mayo Clinic on High Blood Pressure.* Rochester, Minn.: Mayo Clinic, 1999.

> Provides the consumer with information on how to have a longer life while living with high blood pressure. Includes tips on how to prevent high blood pressure, daily menus, a six-step fitness plan, managing medications, issues for women, and home monitoring.

Immune System

Cook, Allan R. *The Immune System Disorders Sourcebook.* Detroit: Omnigraphics, 1997.

> Brings together current information on diseases frequently attributed to immune system failures, including basic information about lupus, multiple sclerosis, Guillain-Barré syndrome, and chronic granulomatous disease. Along with statistical and demographic data and reports on current research initiatives, coverage also includes symptoms, treatments, coping strategies, and current research initiatives for a variety of disorders.

Liver Disease and Related Issues

Bellenir, Karen, ed. *Alcoholism Sourcebook.* Detroit: Omnigraphics, 2000.

> Offers information about the physical and mental consequences of alcohol abuse, including liver disease, pancreatitis, Wernicke-Korsakoff syn-

drome (alcohol dementia), fetal alcohol syndrome, heart disease, kidney disorders, gastrointestinal problems, and immune system compromise.

Turkington, Carol. *Hepatitis C: The Silent Epidemic*. Lincolnwood, Ill.: Contemporary Books, 1998.

According to the foreword, "this book provides a wealth of information in clear, unambiguous language for those who wish to be educated about hepatitis C, for those wishing to know how to prevent acquiring the infection, as well as for those unfortunate enough to be infected. . . . " Chapters include discussions on what hepatitis (all types) is, symptoms, diagnosis, treatment, cirrhosis and other complications, and prevention.

Worman, Howard J. *The Liver Disorders Sourcebook*. Los Angeles: Lowell House, 1999.

A complete guide to the health and care of the liver, *Liver Disorders Sourcebook* includes information on hepatitis, cirrhosis, and liver cancers. Also covers current prevention methods, diagnostic testing and evaluation, and the various treatments available.

Men's Health

Cook, Allan R. *Men's Health Concerns Sourcebook*. Detroit: Omnigraphics, 1998.

Offers information about health issues that affect men, including facts about the top causes of death in men: heart disease, stroke, cancers, prostate disorders, chronic obstructive pulmonary disease, pneumonia and influenza, HIV and AIDS, diabetes, stress, suicide, accidents, and homicides. Also presents facts about such common concerns as impotence, contraception, circumcision, sleep disorders, snoring, hair loss, diet, nutrition, exercise, kidney and urological disorders, and backaches.

Marks, Sheldon. *Prostate and Cancer: A Family Guide to Diagnosis, Treatment and Survival*. Tucson, Ariz.: Fisher Books, 1999.

A revised edition of an earlier text, this title provides information in a question-and-answer format that covers screening and early detection, determining the right treatment, nonsurgical options, support groups, drug therapy (such as Viagra), and recovery.

Nutrition and Exercise

Bellenir, Karen, ed. *Diet and Nutrition Sourcebook*. Detroit: Omnigraphics, 1999.

Offers information on dietary guidelines, including recommended daily intake values, vitamins, minerals, fiber, fat, weight control, dietary supplements, and food additives. Also features special sections on nutritional needs throughout life, and nutrition for people with specific medical concerns such as allergies, high blood cholesterol, hypertension, diabetes, celiac disease, seizure disorders, cancer, and eating disorders. Includes a list of additional resources.

Brody, Jane E., and Reporters of the *New York Times*. *The New York Times Book of Health: How to Feel Fitter, Eat Better, and Live Longer*. New York: Times Books, 1997.

Recognizing that consumers often feel overwhelmed by the relentless stream of health reports, the authors consider current health findings and distill this ocean of often contradictory medical information into a balanced set of sensible guidelines. A compilation of previously published *New York Times* articles, the book is broken down into 11 separate sections.

Gledhill, Kristen M., ed. *Fitness and Exercise Sourcebook*. Detroit: Omnigraphics, 2000.

Offers information about how to begin and maintain a fitness program, fitness as a lifestyle, the link between fitness and diet, advice for specific groups of people, exercise and preexisting medical conditions, and recent research in fitness and exercise. Also includes a glossary and sources of additional information.

Reference

Banerjee, Timir, and Alvaro A. Domingues da Silva, eds. *Signs, Syndromes, and Eponyms: Our Legacy*. Park Ridge. Ill.: American Association of Neurological Surgeons, 1997.

The editors offer a complete description of eponyms in the fields of neurosurgery, neurology, internal medicine, and surgery. The signs and symptoms associated with these disorders are thoroughly described.

Dambro, Mark R., ed. *Griffith's 5-Minute Clinical Consult*. 8th ed. Philadelphia: Lippincott, Williams & Wilkins, 2000.

Covers over 1,000 alphabetically arranged topics that are also cross-indexed by synonyms. This eighth annual edition offers a quick medical reference for current medical diagnosis and treatment.

Davis, Neil M. *Medical Abbreviations: 14,000 Conveniences at the Expense of Communications and Safety*. 9th ed. Huntingdon Valley, Pa.: Neil Davis Associates, 1999.

Probably next to medical terminology itself, deciphering the various abbreviations, acronyms, and symbols is the biggest challenge to consumers. *Medical Abbreviations* offers 14,000 of these puzzles and 20,000 of their possible meanings.

Dorland's Illustrated Medical Dictionary. 29th ed. Philadelphia: W. B. Saunders, 2000.

A core medical dictionary that has kept up with the vast and progressively rapid increase of medical and scientific knowledge since the first edition was published in 1900. According to the preface, the most obvious change in this, the 29th edition is the increase in the number (almost 900) of illustrations and plates as well as the introduction of new terms and concepts.

Everything You Need to Know About Medical Emergencies. Springhouse, Pa.: Springhouse, 1997.

Written by experts in lay language, this book covers what to do in all types of emergencies, including heart attack, stroke, and seizure; broken bones and dislocations; burns and bleeding; breathing difficulties and allergic reactions; poisonings, snakebites, and radiation exposures; head and spinal injuries; sudden blindness and double vision; and a foreign body in the eye, ear, or nose.

Guide to Top Doctors. Washington, D.C.: Center for the Study of Services, 1999.

Lists 15,000 of the top-rated, most highly recommended physicians in America's largest metropolitan areas. Information on each doctor includes details on training, credentials, and office locations. How to get the best care a doctor can provide is also covered.

Handbook of Diagnostic Tests. Springhouse, Pa.: Springhouse, 1999.

Offers information on medical tests, including key diagnostic findings in major disorders, overviews of tests, purpose and indications of tests, patient preparation, procedure and post-test care, precautions, normal findings, abnormal findings, and interfering factors.

Jablonski, Stanley. *Dictionary of Medical Acronyms and Abbreviations*. Philadelphia: Hanley & Belfus, 1998.

Lists acronyms and abbreviations occurring with reasonable frequency in the medical literature as identified through a systematic scanning of medical books and periodicals.

Komaroff, Anthony L. *Harvard Medical School Family Health Guide*. New York: Simon & Schuster, 1999.

This extremely user-friendly health guide helps the consumer answer questions on specific diseases, communicate with doctors, find the best health care, and evaluate health care. It also covers diagnosis, treatment, and prevention of disease in every stage of life. High-quality illustrations are included with symptom charts.

Magalini, Sergio I., and Sabina C. Magalini. *Dictionary of Medical Syndromes*. Philadelphia: Lippincott, Williams & Wilkins, 1997.

Since syndromes are often the most allusive medical topics, this dictionary is a must for any health reference collection. The dictionary format makes it easy for users to find information on difficult-to-find topics.

Margolis, Simeon. *The Johns Hopkins Medical Handbook: The 100 Major Medical Disorders of People Over the Age of 50, Plus a Directory to the Leading Teaching Hospitals, Research Organizations, Treatment Centers, and Support Groups*. New York: Rebus, 1999.

Although many medical encyclopedias are available to the general public, this is the only one that specifically addresses health concerns of people over 50 years of age. The purpose of this encyclopedia is to be a ready reference source rather than to report the most recent advances in the field.

Merck Manual of Medical Information: Home Edition. Whitehouse Station, N.J.: Merck Research Laboratories, 1997.

Published to meet a growing demand by the general public for highly detailed, sophisticated medical information, this is more or less a translation of the *Merck Manual* into lay language. It includes the same information found in the *Merck Manual*, save some of the more technical descriptions that few lay readers would need (such as the exact sounds of heart murmurs or the appearance of diseased tissue under a microscope).

Olendorf, Donna, Christine Jeryan, and Karen Boyden, eds. *The Gale Encyclopedia of Medicine*. Farmington Hills, Mich.: Gale Research, 1999.

According to the introduction, this five-volume set is "a one-stop source for medical information on nearly 1,500 common medical disorders, conditions, tests, and treatments, including high-profile diseases such as AIDS, Alzheimer's disease, cancer, and heart attack." This encyclopedia defines terms in lay language, simplifying the medical jargon so that the consumer can understand.

Tierney, Lawrence M., Stephen J. McPhee, and Maxine A. Papadakis. *Current Medical Diagnosis and Treatment*. New York: Lange Medical Books, 2001.

> Although written for physicians, this can be a valuable reference tool for the more sophisticated health information researcher. Provides information on the latest advances in adult outpatient and inpatient medicine as well as answers to clinical best-practice questions. Covers all areas of internal medicine, gynecology, obstetrics, urology, dermatology, ophthalmology, otolaryngology, psychiatry, neurology, and toxicology.

Respiratory System

Kimball, Chad T., ed. *Colds, Flu and Other Common Ailments Sourcebook*. Detroit: Omnigraphics, 2000.

> Offers information about such ailments as colds, coughs, flu, sinus problems, headaches, fever, nausea and vomiting, menstrual cramps, diarrhea, constipation, hemorrhoids, back pain, dandruff, dry and itchy skin, cuts, scrapes, sprains, and bruises. Also includes information about prevention, self-care, choosing a doctor, over-the-counter medicines, and folk remedies. Has a glossary and a directory of other resources.

Matthews, Dawn D., ed. *Lung Disorders Sourcebook*. Detroit: Omnigraphics, 2000.

> Offers information about emphysema, pneumonia, tuberculosis, asthma, cystic fibrosis, and other lung disorders. Includes facts about diagnostic procedures, treatment strategies, disease prevention efforts, and risk factors (such as smoking, air pollution, and exposure to asbestos, radon, and other agents). Has a glossary and a directory of other resources.

Muth, Annemarie S., ed. *Allergies Sourcebook*. Detroit: Omnigraphics, 2000.

> Offers information about the causes of allergies, including genetic predisposition and early exposure to allergens, as well as triggers (such as pollen, mold, dust mites, ozone, tobacco smoke, formaldehyde, food, insects, animal dander, cosmetics, and medication). Also includes tips on identification, prevention, and treatment, as well as statistical data, a glossary, and resources for further help and information.

Muth, Annemarie S., ed. *Asthma Sourcebook*. Detroit: Omnigraphics, 2000.

> Offers information about asthma (including symptoms), traditional and nontraditional remedies, treatment advances, quality-of-life aids, medical research updates, and the role of allergies, exercise, age, the environment, and genetics in the development of asthma. Also includes statistical data, a glossary, and directories of support groups and other resources.

Young, Stuart H., Bruce S. Dobozin, and Margaret Miner. *Allergies: The Complete Guide to Diagnosis, Treatment, and Daily Management*. New York: Penguin, 1998.

> The authors dispute many myths about allergies and offer long-term help to both the seasonal and the chronic sufferer. This guide helps patients make informed decisions about diagnostic tests, nasal antihistamines, corticosteroid sprays, homeopathic remedies, and emergency relief for severe allergic reactions.

Women's Health

American Medical Association. *Essential Guide to Menopause*. New York: Pocket Books, 1998.

> This AMA book provides information on physical symptoms throughout all phases of menopause; feeling good emotionally; early detection of heart disease, breast cancer, and other health risks; osteoporosis prevention; such treatments as hormone replacement therapy, prescription medications, and complementary therapies; gynecological problems and procedures; lifestyle recommendations for fitness, nutrition, and stress management; and staying sexually active during menopause.

Berger, Karen, and John Bostwick. *A Woman's Decision: Breast Care, Treatment, and Reconstruction*. 3d ed. St. Louis, Mo.: Quality Medical Publishing, 1998.

> With more than 150 photographs and drawings, this third edition details the newest treatments and reconstructive procedures for breast cancer treatment and rehabilitation. Information includes genetic and hormonal therapy, endoscopic surgery, image-guided biopsy, lumpectomy versus mastectomy, skin-sparing mastectomy and immediate reconstruction, and partial reconstruction after lumpectomy.

Carlson, Karen J., Stephanie A. Eisenstat, and Terra Ziporyn. *The Harvard Guide to Women's Health*. Cambridge. Mass.: Harvard University Press, 1996.

> With over 300 entries in an A–Z listing of major disorders, the authors' aim is to answer common questions asked of physicians (such as "Is this normal?" and "Do I need to worry about this?"). The major focus of the guide is on diseases that might affect a woman's reproductive system, such as breast lumps, cervical cancer, endometriosis, ovarian cysts, and sexually transmitted diseases.

Cook, Alan R., ed. *Osteoporosis Sourcebook*. Detroit: Omnigraphics, 2000.

> Offers information about primary and secondary osteoporosis, juvenile osteoporosis, related conditions, and other bone diseases (such as fibrous

dysplasia, myeloma, osteogenesis imperfecta, osteopetrosis, and Paget's disease). Also includes information on risk factors, treatments, and traditional and nontraditional pain management. Has a glossary and a resource directory.

Doran, Annette Thevenin. *Menopause: Questions You Have, Answers You Need*. Allentown, Pa.: People's Medical Society, 1999.
The author provides information on such topics as what a body experiences before, during, and after menopause; how to treat symptoms naturally through diet, nutrition, and exercise; how to prevent and treat menopause-related health conditions; what the benefits and risks of hormone replacement therapy are; and what alternative therapies are available.

Hudson, Tori. *Women's Encyclopedia of Natural Medicine: Alternative Therapies and Integrative Medicine*, Lincolnwood, Ill.: Contemporary Publishing Group, 1999.
Written to help women make informed decisions on combining conventional and alternative medicine, this guide discusses the use of alternative therapies for many female health concerns, including cancer prevention, contraception, heart conditions, and sexually transmitted diseases. Coverage includes vitamin supplements, herbs, diet, bodywork, and exercise.

Lane, Nancy E. *The Osteoporosis Book: A Guide for Patients and Their Families*. New York: Oxford University Press, 1999.
Helps readers make informed healthcare choices that will both reduce the risk of osteoporosis and enhance the quality of life. The author provides information on medical breakthroughs that allow doctors to predict more accurately who is at risk of osteoporosis, helps readers evaluate their own risk factors, provides practical advice on coping with osteoporosis, and guides patients in safeguarding against further deterioration.

Marti, James. *Holistic Pregnancy and Childbirth*. See the section "Complementary and Alternative Medicine" earlier in this chapter.

Mayer, Musa. *Advanced Breast Cancer: A Guide to Living with Metastatic Disease*. See the section "Cancer" earlier in this chapter.

Notelovitz, Morris. *Stand Tall: Every Woman's Guide to Preventing and Treating Osteoporosis*. Gainesville, Fla.: Triad Publishing, 1998.
A practical, comprehensive guide to osteoporosis, this book covers such topics as detecting bone loss, diagnosis, therapies for prevention, and treatment.

Prucha, Edward J., ed. *Breast Cancer Sourcebook*. Detroit: Omnigraphics, 2000.
> Offers information about breast cancer, including diagnostic methods, treatment options, alternative therapies, self-help information, related health concerns, statistical and demographic data, and facts for men with breast cancer. Coverage includes statistical and demographic data, treatment options, and strategies for coping. Has a glossary and a directory of further resources.

Prucha, Edward J., ed. *Cancer Sourcebook for Women*. Detroit: Omnigraphics, 2000.
> Offers information about specific forms of cancer that affect women, including cervical cancer, ovarian cancer, endometrial cancer, uterine sarcoma, vaginal cancer, vulvar cancer, and gestational trophoblastic tumor. Coverage includes statistical information and facts about tests and treatments. Has a glossary and a list of additional resources.

Slupik, Ramona I., and Kathleen Cahill Allison. *American Medical Association Complete Guide to Women's Health*. New York: Random House, 1996.
> Although this book is a little old, it is an authoritative, reliable, and comprehensive guide for every stage of a woman's life. Includes information on such pressing health concerns as heart disease, cancer, osteoporosis, sexually transmitted diseases, stress, and depression. Includes over 700 illustrations, graphs, and charts, as well as a color atlas of the body, practical guides, symptoms charts, and a list of common questions women ask.

Wallis, Lila A., and Marian Betancourt. *The Whole Woman: Take Charge of Your Health in Every Phase of Your Life*. New York: Avon Books, 1999.
> Each section of this book deals with a different chronological phase of a woman's life, outlining specific health conditions unique to women during these phases. These phases include adolescence, the adult woman, the perimenopausal years, and the postmenopausal years. According to the authors, the book was written as a guide for women so that they can "enter into a partnership with their physicians and health care providers."

Miscellaneous

Caldwell, Wilma. *Obesity Sourcebook*. Detroit: Omnigraphics, 2000.
> Provides information about diseases and other problems associated with obesity, including facts about risk factors, prevention issues, and management approaches. Also includes statistical and demographic informa-

tion, information about special populations, research updates, a glossary, and a list of additional resources.

Hagen, Philip T., ed. *Mayo Clinic Guide to Self-Care: Answers for Everyday Health Problems.* Rochester, Minn.: Mayo Clinic, 1997.

> Provides practical, easy-to-understand information on more than 150 common medical conditions and issues relating to health. The general sections of the book are "Urgent Care," "General Symptoms," "Common Problems," "Specific Conditions," "Mental Health," "Staying Healthy," "Your Health and the Workplace," "The Healthy Consumer," "Children and Adolescent Health," and "A Few Words About How We Speak."

Henderson, Helene. *Domestic Violence and Child Abuse Sourcebook.* Detroit: Omnigraphics, 2000.

> Offers essential information about the physical, emotional, and sexual abuse of spouses/partners, children, and elders. Also discusses stalking and teen dating violence, and includes information about hotlines, safe houses, and safety plans as well as a directory of other resources.

Hunder, Gene G., ed. *Mayo Clinic on Arthritis.* Rochester, Minn.: Mayo Foundation for Medical Education and Research, 1998.

> Sponsored by the Mayo Clinic, this book focuses on the two most common types of arthritis—osteoarthritis and rheumatoid arthritis. Information includes guides to the most effective treatments, illustrated exercises, alternative therapies, weight management, easier ways to cook, and how to enjoy travel and recreation.

Kalb, Rosalind C. *Multiple Sclerosis: A Guide for Families.* New York: Demos Vermande, 1998.

> Serves families of multiple sclerosis patients as a guide to strengthening coping skills, finding information on the disease and its ramifications, and making important life decisions. Chapters address cognitive and emotional issues, caregiving, life planning, general health and well-being, and supportive and educational resources.

Kimball, Chad. *Workplace Health and Safety Sourcebook.* Detroit: Omnigraphics, 2000.

> Offers information on musculoskeletal injuries, occupational carcinogens and other toxic materials, child labor, workplace violence, and transmission of HIV and hepatitis viruses. Gives special coverage of such specific industries as mining, agriculture, construction, electrical work, and the medical professions. Also includes statistical information, preventive

measures, ways of reducing stress, a glossary, and a list of additional resources.

Massimini, Kathy, ed. *Genetic Disorders Sourcebook*. Detroit: Omnigraphics, 2000.
Offers information on hereditary diseases and disorders, including cystic fibrosis, Down's syndrome, hemophilia, Huntington's disease, and sickle cell anemia. Also includes information about genes, gene therepy, genetic screening, ethics of gene testing, and genetic counseling. Has a glossary and a resource list.

Matthews, Dawn D., ed. *Eating Disorders Sourcebook*. Detroit: Omnigraphics, 2000.
Offers information on anorexia nervosa, bulimia nervosa, binge eating, food addiction, body dysmorphic disorder, pica, laxative abuse, and night eating syndrome. Also includes information on causes, adverse affects, treatment, and prevention issues. Has a glossary and a list of further resources.

Shannon, Joyce Brennfleck, ed. *Caregiving Sourcebook*. Detroit: Omnigraphics, 2000.
Offers information for caregivers, including a profile of caregivers, a list of caregiving responsibilities, tips for specific conditions, care environments, and the effects of caregivers. Coverage includes legal issues, financial concerns, future planning. Has a glossary and a list of additional resources.

Shannon, Joyce Brennfleck, ed. *Medical Tests Sourcebook*. Detroit: Omnigraphics, 1999.
Offers information on medical tests, including periodic health exams, general screening tests, tests consumers can do at home, x-ray and other radiological tests, electrical tests, tests of blood and other bodily fluids and tissues, scope tests, lung tests, genetic tests, pregnancy screening tests, newborn screening tests, sexually transmitted diseases tests, and computer-aided diagnoses. Also included are a section on paying for medical tests, a glossary, and a list of additional resources.

Shannon, Joyce Brennfleck, ed. *Traveler's Health Sourcebook*. Detroit: Omnigraphics, 2000.
Offers information for travelers, including physical and medical preparations, transportation health and safety, essential information about food and water, sun exposure, insect and snake bites, camping and wilderness

medicine, and travel with physical or medical disabilities. Also includes international travel tips, vaccination recommendations, geographical health issues, disease risks, a glossary, and a list of additional resources.

Shapiro, Randall T. *Symptom Management in Multiple Sclerosis*. New York: Demos Medical Publishing Co., 1998.

The author, a physician who specializes in multiple sclerosis, offers advice on management of the symptoms of the disease, with an emphasis on medical, rehabilitative, and psychological approaches. Chapters include information on fatigue, spasticity, weakness, tremor, walking, sexuality, bladder and bowel symptoms, pain, speech difficulties, swallowing difficulties, cognition, vision problems, dizziness and vertigo, pressure sores, weight gain, numbness, cold feet, and swollen ankles.

Weatherford, M. Lisa, ed. *Plastic Surgery Sourcebook*. Detroit: Omnigraphics, 2000.

Offers information on cosmetic and reconstructive plastic surgery, including statistical information about surgical procedures, things to consider prior to surgery, techniques and tools, emotional and psychological considerations, and procedure-specific information. Also includes a glossary and a list of additional resources.

Weatherford, M. Lisa, ed. *Podiatry Sourcebook*. Detroit: Omnigraphics, 2000. Includes information about foot conditions, diseases, and injuries, including bunions, corns, calluses, athlete's foot, plantar warts, hammertoes and clawtoes, club foot, heel pain, and gout. Also presents facts about foot care, disease prevention, foot safety, and choosing a foot-care specialist. Includes a glossary and a list of additional resources.

6

Recommended Consumer Health Resources About and For Children

When it comes to consumer health and children, there are two kinds of information: consumer health information about children and consumer health information for children.

Consumer Health Information About Children

Parents seeking information relating to the health of their children frequently turn to libraries for answers. Such parental queries can range from routine requests for information about child wellness to desperate pleas for "everything you have" on some life-threatening disease or condition. Fear and guilt can make parents demanding customers—which is not to say that concerned parents do not deserve the same service and access to information accorded everyone else. The following print and electronic resources can help provide parents (and other caretakers of children) with quality consumer health information.

Print Resources

There are thousands of books having to do with children's health, many of which focus on specific diseases or conditions. The books listed below are all general in focus and, while they are not a complete collection in themselves, could form the nucleus of an up-to-date pediatric consumer health reference section.

Feldman, William, ed. *The 3 A.M. Handbook: The Most Commonly Asked Questions About Your Child's Health*. New York: Facts on File, 1998.
> Written in question-and-answer format by a team of pediatricians, *The 3 A.M. Handbook* is a practical guide that includes such chapters as "Choosing Your Child's Doctor," "Spitting Up: Vomiting and Diarrhea," "Research: Being Part of the Picture," and "Emergency First Aid." Includes illustrations and lists of support and information groups. Indexed.

Friedman, Alan H., et al. *Complete Directory for Pediatric Disorders*. Lakeville, Conn.: Grey House, 2000.
> For each of the dozens of pediatric disorders it covers, *Complete Direc-*

tory for Pediatric Disorders provides a thorough description followed by information about related associations, support groups, Web sites, newsletters, pamphlets, children's books, and research centers. Other sections of *Complete Directory* include "General Resources," "The Human Body," and "Guidelines for Obtaining Additional Information and Resources." Includes three indexes (Entry, Geographic, and Subject) as well as a medical glossary.

Gallin, Pamela, and Kathy Matthews. *Savvy Mom's Guide to Medical Care: Everything You Need to Know to Get Top Quality Care for Your Child from One of the Nation's Leading Physicians.* New York: St. Martin's Press, 1999.
    Coauthored by a pediatrician/mother and billed as "what your best friend would tell you if she were a pediatrician," *Savvy Mom's Guide* is an insider's look at the world of pediatric health care. Reassuring yet eminently practical, this guide aims to make parents into informed advocates for their children's health. Includes such helpful tips as the best time of day to schedule a doctor's appointment for your child, the best way to get a child to take medicine, and what to do during medical emergencies.

Schiff, Donald, and Steven P. Shelov. *Guide to Your Child's Symptoms: The Official, Complete Home Reference, Birth Through Adolescence.* New York: Villard, 1999.
    A publication of the American Academy of Pediatrics, *Guide to Your Child's Symptoms* is divided into sections based on a child's age and then further subdivided into specific symptoms. Using this book parents can quickly determine possible causes of—and appropriate actions to take in response to—their child's symptoms. Includes an illustrated first-aid and safety guide. Indexed.

Schmitt, Barton D., and J. Todd Jacobs. *Instructions for Pediatric Patients.* 2d ed. Philadelphia: Saunders, 1999.
    Instructions for Pediatric Patients is a book of model instructions intended to be duplicated and handed out by pediatricians to the parents of sick children. Though the instructions have undergone careful scientific peer review, they are written in easy-to-understand language. The instructions address most of the common health problems of children.

Schwartz, M. William, and Bruce Goldfarb. *The 5 Minute Child Health Advisor.* Baltimore: Lippincott, Williams & Wilkins, 1998.
    Provides concise but essential information on over 150 childhood diseases and conditions. Each entry is divided into "Basics" (descriptions, signs and symptoms, causes, and scope), "Diagnosis," "Treatment," "Medications," "Follow-Up," and "Common Questions and Answers." Includes a section of medical definitions. Indexed.

Traisman, Edward S., Karen Judy, Mary Jane Staba, Donna Kotulak, Dennis Connaughton. *American Medical Association Complete Guide to Your Children's Health*. New York: Random House, 1999.

> The heart of this book is a comprehensive encyclopedia containing information on hundreds of topics related to children's health. Also includes two major sections ("Your Healthy Child from Birth Through Adolescence" and "Caring for Your Child's Health") as well as decision trees that help parents respond appropriately to whatever symptoms their child exhibits. Copiously illustrated. Indexed.

Wootan, George. *Take Charge of Your Child's Health: A Parents' Guide to Recognizing Symptoms and Treating Minor Illnesses at Home*. 2d ed. New York: Marlowe, 2000.

> *Take Charge of Your Child's Health* includes such features as a section on childhood allergies, questions to ask the pediatrician, instructions on how to do a physical examination, and the 13 signs of a sick child. The author, a pediatrician, is a strong advocate of the idea that parents should play an active role in the care of their children's health, and some of his ideas are controversial. Indexed.

Zand, Janet, Rachel Walton, and Bob Rountree. *Smart Medicine for a Healthier Child: A Practical A-to-Z Reference to Natural and Conventional Treatments for Infants and Children*. Garden City Park, N.Y.: Avery Publishing Group, 1994.

> There are hundreds of books about alternative medicine for children. Many of these are polemical, and a few are downright dangerous. The virtue of *Smart Medicine* is that its authors—a natural-medicine practitioner, a traditionally licensed doctor, and a pediatric nurse—take a balanced approach that offers parents a full range of options rather than dogma. Covers most of the common childhood ailments.

Electronic Resources

Thousands of Web sites provide information about children's health. The handful of Web sites that follow are listed here because they

- Focus on children's health
- Provide a good quantity of quality information or links
- Provide or point to information on a broad range of children's health topics

Children's Hospitals in North America
www.library.tmc.edu/childrenshospital.html

...st information about children's health is found on Web
...d and maintained by children's hospitals. The **Children's**
...**North America** Web page is a good starting point for finding
...hospitals on the Web. Links are arranged by name of the hos-
...well as by state/province. Note that many of these Web sites also
...de excellent consumer health information *for* children.

...en's Virtual Hospital
...w.vh.org/VCH

Produced by the University of Iowa, the strength of **Children's Virtual Hospital** is "Common Problems in Pediatrics," a section that provides both parents and healthcare providers with in-depth information on nearly 50 childhood ailments. Each document in **Children's Virtual Hospital** includes information regarding authorship, peer-review status, date of creation, and date of last revision.

Facts for Families and Other Resources
www.aacap.org/info_families

Produced by the American Academy of Child and Adolescent Psychiatry, **Facts for Families and Other Resources** is the leading online source for consumer health information about developmental, emotional, behavioral, and mental disorders in children and adolescents. Within **Facts for Families** consumers will find peer-reviewed publications produced (in both English and Spanish) by the American Academy of Child and Adolescent Psychiatry. Topics covered range from "Manic Depression" to "Helping Your Teen Become a Safe Driver" to "Know Your Health Insurance Benefits." All the **Facts for Families** publications are dated, and the entire collection is searchable by keyword.

KidsHealth for Parents
www.kidshealth.org/parent

A service of the Nemours Foundation, **KidsHealth for Parents** provides information on such topics as "General Health," "Emotions & Behavior," "Pregnancy & Newborns," "Positive Parenting," and "Medical Problems." A "Newsroom" section keeps parents informed on the latest developments in children's health.

Medem: Medical Library: Children's Health
www.medem.com

A joint venture founded by seven leading national medical specialty societies, **Medem: Medical Library: Children's Health** provides access to hundreds of publications covering just about every aspect of childhood health.

Most of these publications bear the imprint of the American Academy of Pediatrics, though other medical associations are represented as well. Each publication is rated according to its complexity so that users know up front if they will be dealing with "Introductory Health Info," "General Health Info," "Advanced Resources," or "Professional/Research." The entire library is searchable by keyword.

You and Your Family
www.aap.org/family

Produced especially for healthcare consumers, **You and Your Family** provides a wealth of up-to-date information from the well-respected and proactive American Academy of Pediatrics. One highlight of **You and Your Family** is "The Pediatric Internet: Reviews of Internet Resources by AAP Fellows." Although some of the resources linked to on "The Pediatric Internet" provide professional, rather than consumer health, information, every resource has been reviewed by a pediatrician and meets the following criteria for inclusion: usefulness to pediatric practice, substantial, original content, freedom from commercial influence, clearly identified contacts, and accessibility.

Consumer Health Information for Children

Children seek consumer health information for a variety of reasons. They may want to learn about diseases or conditions afflicting themselves, siblings, parents, or friends. They may be doing research for a school paper or science fair project. Or they may simply be curious. Whatever their motivation, the following resources can help children find answers to their health-related questions.

Print Resources

Finding current consumer health information for children in printed format is a surprisingly hit-or-miss business. A few topics, such as nutrition and cancer, are perennially well represented in print literature for children, while the availability of books on hot topics (these currently include death and dying, smoking, and eating disorders) comes and goes. For many other health-related topics, however, the pickings for children can be more miss than hit, especially if current information is wanted.

One way to determine if there is a current children's book covering a particular disease or condition is to search WorldCat (the OCLC database) using the term "juvenile literature" *plus* a relevant keyword *plus* a date limit. Another approach is to consult one of the printed subject guides to nonfiction children's literature, such as *Beacham's Guide to Literature for Young Adults,*[1] *Middle and Junior High School Library Catalog,*[2] and *Senior High School Library Catalog.*[3]

The following list consists of current print works for children that treat the topic of health broadly rather than focusing on a specific disease or condition. Taken together, these books can fulfill, or at least start to fulfill, just about any child's need for health-related information.

Columbia University's Health Education Program Staff. *The "Go Ask Alice" Book of Answers: A Guide to Good Physical, Sexual and Emotional Health.* New York: Henry Holt, 1998.

> A collection of questions and answers selected from the **Go Ask Alice!** Web site (see the entry under "Electronic Resources" below), this book offers an alternative for those who cannot access that Web site—those who do not have Internet access as well as those whose access to **Go Ask Alice!** is blocked by filtering software.

Darling, David. *The Health Revolution: Surgery and Medicine in the Twenty-First Century.* Parsippany, N.J.: Silver Burdett, 1999.

> Through text and illustrations, *The Health Revolution* catalogs recent advances in medical technology. A good source for children working on homework projects as well as for kids with a more personal interest in the workings of such things as MRIs and microsurgical instruments. Intended for readers in fifth grade and above.

Hyde, Margaret O., and Elizabeth Held Forsyth. *The Disease Book: A Kid's Guide.* New York: Walker, 1997.

> Describes the causes, symptoms, effects, and treatment of a number of diseases and disorders. *The Disease Book* is organized by type of ailment (for example, "Disorders of the Digestive System" and "Mental Illness"). Illustrated. Includes a bibliography and index.

Kowalski, Kathiann M. *Alternative Medicine: Is It for You?* Springfield, N.J.: Enslow, 1998.

> *Alternative Medicine: Is It for You?* lays out the major areas of alternative medicine, explains the difference between alternative and conven-

---

1. *Beacham's Guide to Literature for Young Adults.* Detroit, MI: Gale Group, 1989.
2. Price, Anne, and Juliette Yakov. *Middle and Junior High School Library Catalog.* 8th ed. New York: H. W. Wilson, 2000.
3. Juliette Yakov. *Senior High School Library Catalog.* 15th ed. New York: H. W. Wilson, 1997.

tional medicine, and discusses such related topics as medical fraud and research into alternative therapies. This balanced treatment allows young readers to come to their own conclusions about alternative medicine. Includes an index, glossary, and a selective bibliography. For middle school readers and up.

Newton, David E. *Sick! Diseases and Disorders, Injuries and Infections.* Detroit: UXL, 1999.
> An alphabetical dictionary of ailments, *Sick!* provides a short definition for each entry then follows up with more detailed information about causes, diagnosis, treatments, prevention, and so on. Some attention is paid to alternative therapies. For sixth-grade readers and up.

Olendorf, Donna, Christine Jeryan, and Karen Boyden, eds. *Gale Encyclopedia of Medicine.* 5 vols. Detroit: Gale Research, 1999.
> Though written at too high a level for elementary school students, *Gale Encyclopedia of Medicine* is the closest thing there is to a current, comprehensive encyclopedia of medicine for children. The encyclopedia's approximately 1,500 entries and over 600 illustrations provide information on hundreds of diseases, conditions, medical tests, medical procedures, treatments, and therapies. Includes cross-references, a general index, bibliographies, and contact information for organizations and support groups.

Rattenbury, Jeanne. *Understanding Alternative Medicine.* New York: Franklin Watts, 1999.
> Children, too, are interested in alternative medicine. *Understanding Alternative Medicine* provides young readers with information about systems of alternative medicine (for example, chiropractic, Chinese, and osteopathic) as well as about specific alternative therapies. Written for middle school readers and above. Includes bibliographic references and an index.

Electronic Resources

Consumer Health for Kids
www.nnlm.nlm.nih.gov/scr/conhlth/chforkids2.htm
> Provides annotated links to over 20 major Web sites that provide consumer health information for children. Compiled and maintained by the National Network of Libraries of Medicine, South Central Region.

Go Ask Alice!

www.goaskalice.columbia.edu/

Produced by Columbia University's Health Education Program, **Go Ask Alice!** provides answers to health-related questions submitted anonymously by visitors to the Web site. Major sections of this Web site include "General Health," "Relationships," "Sexuality," "Sexual Health," "Emotional Health," "Fitness & Nutrition," and "Alcohol, Nicotine, & Other Drugs." The sexual nature of many of the questions, as well as the frankness of the answers, has made **Go Ask Alice!** controversial. (It is a favorite target of talk-radio personality "Dr. Laura.") Though the quality of the information provided is first rate, some will be offended by the content of this Web site.

Government Sites for Kids

www.westga.edu/~library/depts/govdoc/kids.shtml

Within its "Health" and "Safety" categories, **Government Sites for Kids** links to over two dozen major U.S. government Web sites that provide children with consumer health information. Linked Web sites range from the National Cancer Institute's **KidsHome** to the National Highway Traffic Safety Administration's **Safety City**.

KidsHealth

kidshealth.org/kid

A service of the Nemours Foundation, KidsHealth provides age-appropriate information on a wide variety of health topics. Its "People, Places, & Things That Help Me" section covers such topics as "Going to the Dentist," "What Happens in the Operating Room," and "What Medicines Are and How They Work." A section called "Word! A Glossary of Medical Terms" defines almost 200 terms. A "Kids' Talk" section answers kids' questions about their bodies and health, and a "Game Closet" makes it fun to learn about health.

MEDLINE*plus*: Children's Page

www.nlm.nih.gov/medlineplus/childrenspage.html

Provides links to child-oriented health information. As with all information on **MEDLINE*plus***, the information on **Children's Page** must meet the **MEDLINE*plus* Selection Guidelines** (*www.nlm.nih.gov/medlineplus/criteria.html*). Categories covered include "General/Overviews," "Anatomy/Physiology," "Nutrition," "Prevention/Screening," and "Specific Conditions/Aspects."

TeensHealth

www.kidshealth.org/teen/

Also a service of the Nemours Foundation, **TeensHealth** uses a format similar to that of **KidsHealth** to provide age-appropriate health information for teenagers. Major sections include "Body Basics," "Sexual Health," "Q & A," and "Health Problems."

PART III

Consumer Health Services for Libraries

7
Creating Consumer Healthcare Services

There are many reasons why consumers increasingly search for health information. First, and probably foremost, is the fact that as managed health care becomes more prevalent, patients are forced to take more responsibility in managing their own health care. Many consumers are finding that it is taking longer to make a doctor's appointment and, once in the office, they get less time with their doctor. In addition, pharmaceutical companies have begun marketing directly to the consumer, bypassing health professionals and spurring consumers into a more active role in learning about, and requesting from their doctors, medications they believe will help them. Finally, educated consumers are becoming generally less hesitant about challenging decisions made by a health professional and/or seeking out alternative health choices.

Where Do Consumers Find Health Information?

Consumers are finding health information by many means, including:

- Visiting public and medical libraries
- Searching the Internet
- Reading self-help books and consumer health magazines
- Contacting associations through toll-free phone numbers
- Asking friends and relatives who have encountered similar problems
- E-mailing addresses found on specific health Web sites
- Receiving information through the media, since television, radio, and the print media all have health information programs
- Identifying chat groups or listservs comprised of people with similar health concerns

Not surprisingly, consumers are finding that health information is becoming more readily available on the Internet. One of the first moves to make health information accessible to the consumer came in 1996 when Vice President Al Gore announced that federal agencies would make health information freely available through the Internet. The National Library of Medicine (NLM) was one of the first agencies to move in this direction by making access to the MEDLINE database available through **PubMed** (*www.ncbi.nlm.nih.gov/entrez/query.fcgi*). This database was followed in 1998 with **MEDLINE***plus* (*www.medlineplus.gov/*), the consumer-based Web site. The U.S. Department of Health and Human Services followed suit with **healthfinder** (*www. healthfinder.gov/*). Around this same time, a joint project of multiple institutions in metropolitan New York launched **NOAH** (*www.noah-health.org/*) and a similar consortium in Ohio created **NetWellness** (*www.netwellness. org/*). In 1999 NLM launched another valuable database, **ClinicalTrials.gov** (*www.clinicaltrials.gov*) to help consumers locate valuable clinical trials on specific diseases and conditions.

Whether because or in spite of the huge amounts of health information available on the Internet, many consumers find their way to academic medical and hospital libraries. There the health information they encounter is often written in language aimed at those with many years of health education—doctors, nurses, and physician assistants, for example. Taking note of the increasing interest in consumer health information, many medical and hospital libraries have begun collecting consumer health information as well as information aimed at healthcare professionals. In many cases, costs for such materials have been offset by private or grant funds, so as to not deplete the money put into the ever-growing cost of maintaining a professional medical collection. Even though many medical and hospital libraries are making an effort to reach consumers, such libraries are typically located in medical centers or in hospitals where consumers can find it difficult, or even intimidating, to visit. For example, although the Houston Academy of Medicine–Texas Medical Center (HAM–TMC) Library has been purchasing consumer health materials for about three years and employs a librarian dedicated to serving consumers, few consumers visit the library. Located among the Texas Medical Center's 42 institutions (13 of which are hospitals), the HAM–TMC Library is hard to find, parking is expensive, and many consumers assume that the library is open only to Texas Medical Center personnel. It is the brave consumer who ventures from home, doctor's office, or loved one's bedside to visit the library. Because HAM–TMC Library reference staff have found that many consumers seek information by phone or by contacting the consumer librarian via e-mail, HAM–TMC Library has undertaken marketing efforts to bring more consumers into the building.

Since medical and hospital libraries can seem intimidating, consumers are more likely to seek healthcare information in a place where they have always felt comfortable—the public library. However, public librarians can be intimidated by health questions because they feel they lack the information resources or experience to help answer complicated health questions. As a librarian from the Houston Public Library once said, "public librarians are generalists by nature. It is difficult to become an expert in any particular subject area." Because of these problems, public and medical librarians are finding it beneficial to work together—and learn from each other—to help serve this important client group. For example, medical librarians can teach the public librarians to search the basic health information databases and sites such as **PubMed**, **MEDLINE***plus*, and **healthfinder**. Public librarians can help the medical librarians by teaching them how to market library services and how to serve clients with low literacy levels or limited English-language skills.

Collaboration Between Public and Medical Libraries

As more people begin to search for health information, one of the best things that libraries can do is collaborate on projects to help serve healthcare consumers. In 1998 NLM sponsored a pilot project partnering selected academic medical libraries with public libraries, in an effort to determine the informational needs of health consumers and to help train public librarians to better help health information consumers. The HAM–TMC Library partnered with the Houston Public Library (HPL) on one of these pilot projects. During the course of the project the HAM–TMC Library staff trained almost all the adult reference librarians in the 35-branch HPL system to search the major health databases and sites. During the training, the public librarians were given a tour of the Jesse H. Jones Community Health Information Service, shown the major reference sources used at the HAM–TMC Library reference desk, and encouraged to refer any clients they could not help to the medical library. Simultaneously, the HPL librarians kept records of the types of health-related questions that were being asked and reported these findings back to NLM. The project was so successful that the staff of the nearby Harris County Public Library (which serves areas of the county not located in the Houston city limits) asked if their adult reference staff could also be trained. This pilot project has begun a partnership that still continues, with each library trying to find the best methods to help the healthcare consumers of the city of Houston and of Harris County.

The Briscoe Library at the University of Texas Health Sciences Center in San Antonio conducted a similar project. Instead of partnering with one public library, however, they partnered with the state-supported Alamo Area Library System and reached out to eight public libraries in the rural areas surrounding their large urban area. At the end of these two projects, both libraries reported similar experiences to NLM, even though one medical library worked primarily with branch libraries in a major metropolitan area while the other worked primarily with small, rural public libraries.[1]

Findings of the projects included the following:

- Public libraries are a valuable resource for consumer health information

---

1. Tobia, Rajia, and Deborah Halsted. "Medical Questions Pilot Project Update." *Network News* 44 (September/October 1999): pp. 1, 4.

because often they are more accessible to the general public. Many people are intimidated by large medical centers and medical libraries and feel more comfortable visiting their neighborhood libraries. In many communities, particularly those that are small or rural, the public library may be the only library available for answering health questions.

- Some consumers may feel conspicuous visiting their local librarian (whom they might have known for many years) to discuss personal health problems, such as AIDS or sexually transmitted diseases. In this case, the consumer might feel more comfortable visiting a larger academic medical library where they can remain anonymous.
- Public libraries purchase health-related books that are written at the level of the general public. Academic medical libraries typically purchase materials written for health professionals. Most consumers seeking health information have difficulty understanding technical materials.
- Healthcare consumers want access to information immediately and for free. They are not willing to wait or pay for articles and books obtained through such means as interlibrary loan.
- Since public librarians need to know how to find information on many different topics, training by a medical librarian to find health information is beneficial. Unfortunately, since many public libraries are understaffed, it can be difficult to find time to attend training. Follow-up training is also important, as the ways of accessing health information change rapidly.
- Many public libraries have a limited number of Internet-connected computers, so once staff have been trained, computers may not be readily available for them to practice the newly learned skills. For example, many of the small public libraries participating in the San Antonio project had, at the time, only one computer for both public and staff use.[2]
- Public libraries have a long history of outreach to their communities. Academic medical librarians can learn a lot from their public library colleagues about marketing library programs and services.

As a result of these public library/medical library pilot projects, NLM has extended the National Network of Libraries of Medicine (NN/LM) consumer health outreach projects through its regional NN/LM network. The eight Regional Medical Libraries located in various geographic areas of the United States have money available for Partners for Access to Consumer Health Information Program (PACHI). Contact your local Regional Medical Library by calling (800) 338–7657. Many state libraries have worked to get all their

---

2. Some of these libraries used project funds provided by the NLM to purchase one or two more computers. Those that did so also had to find ways or funds to connect this equipment to the Internet.

public libraries connected to the Internet. Many have also secured statewide licensing for such databases as *Health Reference Center* for all public libraries in their states so that consumers can access this full-text information at the public library. Progressive public libraries have designed password-protected remote access systems, so that databases like *Health Reference Center* can be accessed from the home, office, or anywhere else.

Basic Health Reference

Typically, healthcare consumers are patients, members of a patient's family, or caregivers (who may also be family members). These patrons are not all that different from anyone else approaching a reference desk seeking an answer to a question. Although the information requested by a healthcare consumer may be specialized and include unfamiliar, multisyllabic words, librarians must conduct a traditional in-depth reference interview to ascertain exactly what the true reference question might be. One major difference between a general reference question and a health-related question is that the reference interview may take longer because:

- The sensitive nature of many health questions means that, compared to asking a general question, consumers might have a more difficult time formulating the real question.
- Many health terms and concepts are as unfamiliar to the reference librarian as they are to the healthcare consumer.
- More often than with other patrons, healthcare consumers may have low literacy levels, not speak English, be aged, have a handicap (such as hearing impairment or loss of vision) or be distraught in the wake of a disturbing diagnosis.

One way to make healthcare consumers more comfortable during a reference interview is to provide a private area for such transactions. Recognizing that reference interviews concerning health problems such as AIDS or hepatitis C are of a sensitive nature, the HAM–TMC Library set up a separate area containing the consumer monographic collection and an Internet computer. At the outset of the service, this setup seemed to be ideal. As the program progressed, the consumer health librarian found that the solitary computer is mostly used for non-consumer health purposes. Additionally, the consumer health librarian found that consumers still hesitate to talk about their health concerns in this small open reading room because others use the tables to study. For this reason she has requested a separate interview room, with a door and walls, to conduct the more sensitive interviews. For libraries that lack the space for a separate consumer health area or interview room, conducting such interviews in a private staff office is one option.

Malpractice and Liability

Information malpractice and liability are matters of concern when providing medical information to consumers. Any librarian offering health information must be careful to offer only the information provided by the sources consulted and never to help interpret this information. For example, if someone calls asking for side effects of a particular drug, the librarian must read exactly from the source—such as the *Physicians' Desk Reference*—and not offer any advice based on personal experience. The librarian may act as an information provider but never as a healthcare provider. If for some reason a healthcare consumer has an ill effect from the information given, the liability could fall on the librarian if information was not provided exactly as presented in the printed source or database. Often, healthcare consumers ask a librarian to refer them to a doctor who treats a specific illness or condition. Again, it is not the librarian's place to make such referrals. Most states and large urban areas have medical societies that maintain databases of what doctors in the area treat specific conditions.

Consider the following example of a healthcare consumer seeking inappropriate assistance from a librarian. An elderly woman telephoned asking for help for her son, a military veteran who received his health care through the local Veterans Affairs Medical Center. The woman was distraught, saying that the VA doctors were killing her son and couldn't the librarian help find someone who could treat him for free. The woman also wanted the librarian to interpret her son's medical records, which she tried to read over the phone. She was certain that some book in the library would help the librarian do this. The librarian explained to the woman that she could not recommend another doctor, that perhaps the local medical society could and provided the number. When it came to interpreting the records, the librarian explained that she was not a health professional and that the woman would need to come into the library herself and do some research. The woman responded that she was disabled and could not leave her house. The librarian did try to calm the woman, got her address, and mailed her some basic information taken from a consumer health information database.

While some people want more help than librarians can give, there are those healthcare consumers who are content to do research on their own. An elderly man frequently visited a medical library, always bringing along his comatose, wheelchair-bound wife. Never bothering anyone, the man only used a computer in the reference area, typing with his right hand as he held his wife's hand in his left hand. As staff walked by, it became obvious that the man was looking for health information. After the first visit, the consumer librarian stopped by to ask the man if there was anything she could do to help in his search for information, explaining that she did not want to interfere if he was comfortable he was finding the best information. He explained his wife's con-

dition and said that he was looking for a clinical trial for her. He was qu.
aware of the proper databases, he just needed access to a computer with Internet
access. The librarian told him that he was welcome to use the computer any
time and to please call her if he needed help.

It is a good practice for a library to provide a disclaimer with any printed
health information it makes available to the public. As an example, the disclaimer on the *Houston HealthWays* site (*http://hhw.library.tmc.edu*) states:

> Not all sources of electronic information—including those found on
> the Internet—provide information that is current, accurate, or com-
> plete. The people and organizations that bring you Houston
> HealthWays cannot control or monitor the content of electronic in-
> formation. Users of Houston HealthWays must exercise critical judg-
> ment when evaluating any information. Health-care information
> found on the Internet—or through any other print or electronic re-
> source—is not a substitute for a professional medical opinion. Any-
> one with a medical problem should contact a qualified medical pro-
> fessional.

The disclaimer found on the **NetWellness** homepage (*www.netwellness.org*)
serves as another good example. It states:

> Only your personal physician or other health professional you con-
> sult can best advise you on matters of your health based on your
> medical history, your family medical history, your medication his-
> tory, and how information from any of these databases may apply
> to you.

Any such a disclaimer should stress to the consumer that information found in
the library, on the Internet, or anywhere else should only supplement, not
replace the expert opinion of a trained health professional.

One very important area where the librarian can help the consumer is in the
identification of quality information. As all know, bad health information can
be harmful or even fatal. Anyone with a little technical experience can mount
a Web page that offers health information, good or bad, and, as explained in
Chapter 5, there is no simple means of separating good health information
from bad. Librarians can be instrumental in directing clients to Web sites that
are most certain to offer quality information. These sites would include those
produced by government agencies (federal, state, county, or city), major health
institutions (such as medical schools), major health associations (such as the
American Medical Associations), and associations dedicated to specific diseases or conditions (such as the American Diabetes Association). Commercial

sites (such as those of pharmaceutical companies) can also offer helpful information, but because these sites are used as marketing tools, their objectivity is suspect. Chapter 5 has information to help librarians evaluate health Web sites and Chapter 6 provides an annotated list of consumer health Web sites.

Progressive libraries might consider creating a Web page (or Web pages) to provide links only to health Web sites of high quality. Such a resource could serve as a starting point for answering health questions. Since Web pages are easily updated, sites could be added as the health information service grows.

Marketing

It has been the experience of the HAM–TMC Library that the popular adage "If you build it, they will come" does not hold true. As mentioned above, we have found that many deterrents keep consumers from entering an academic medical or hospital library. Medical libraries can learn much from their public library colleagues who have been marketing library services for years. Some suggestions include:

- **Send press/news releases of major events to the medical editors for all the local media (television, radio, and print).** Major events could include the kickoff of your consumer health program, acquisition of materials or equipment, general updates on the service, or anything that might catch an editor's eye. Press releases should be short and to the point—no more than one page long if possible. A press release should be written in pyramid format, with the most important information first and the least important information last, and it should answer the questions: who? what? when? where? and why? Do not forget to include a release date so it is clear when the information can be published or announced, and include name plus contact information for key personnel. The text should be double-spaced and printed on only one side of the paper. If it continues beyond one page, type MORE at the bottom of each page. Type ### or –30– at the end of the release to indicate the end of the item. It also helps to have multilingual staff or contacts so that press releases can be submitted to foreign-language media.
- **Hold a press conference for major events.** Tips for handling successful press conferences include:
  — Hold them only for very special event.
  — Start on time.
  — Follow a specific script.
  — Keep the press conference short.
  — Provide a press kit, which should include:
    * A list of materials in the kit
    * A copy of the press release

* A fact sheet about the event or special project
* Relevant photographs
* A list of contact people
* Possibly an institutional annual report
* A business card for your public relations person or library director.

- **Try to partner with local agencies that produce health information for the general public.** Most television stations have health reporters. Contact these reporters personally and offer the library's service in researching health topics. Many hospitals and doctor's offices offer free pamphlets and brochures on common health problems. Work with these people on producing and/or disseminating these materials.

- **Work with local health agencies to produce public service announcements (PSAs) to air either on local television or radio stations.** English- and Spanish-language PSAs for the Houston HealthWays project were produced by the Houston Department of Health and Human Services (HDHHS), a project partner, and they air regularly on the city of Houston's municipal channel. Since HDHHS has its own production department, there was no cost to produce the videos. A local notable Hispanic leader served as the spokesperson. Since he is also a city of Houston employee, there was no charge for his services.

- **Get involved in local health events by setting up a table or booth at local health fairs, marathons, or job fairs.** When electricity and phone/Internet connections are available, bring a laptop computer so that you can show off your own or other consumer health Web sites. If you plan to do many exhibits/health fairs, it is a good idea to design and purchase a tabletop display. This display should include the library's name or the project's name in large letters. Other materials should be attached with Velcro™, so that as technology changes it is easy to change the display.

- **Create inexpensive give-away items to be distributed at classes, health fairs, and exhibits.** For the Houston HealthWays project we designed Rolodex™ cards with the logo, URL, and pertinent phone numbers. These cards are easily printed out on a laser printer. The same design was also used on magnets purchased from a promotional agent.[3]

---

3. If you produce and distribute magnets, it is very important to remind everyone not to stick them to a computer, as they can damage computer memory.

8
Evaluating Consumer Health Resources for Your Users

Two distinct types of evaluation are important to healthcare consumers. One type involves the evaluation of health information; the other, the evaluation of healthcare practitioners and institutions. The chapter concerns itself with both types of evaluation.

Evaluating Health Information

The sheer amount of health information available in print and online makes evaluation difficult; the fact that healthcare decisions can be, literally, life-and-death decisions makes evaluation absolutely necessary.

The first rule of evaluating health information is to approach *all* such information with a healthy (pun intended) skepticism. This goes for both print and electronic information. While bad health information on the Internet tends to draw the most attention, any number of current mass-market magazines and trade books are keeping up their end of this bad bargain, too. Whether bad health information comes in print or electronic form, whether it is generated by con artists, zealots, pranksters, bad scientists, the misinformed, or harried journalists trying to churn out copy, it can harm the unwary. Bad information can cause them to:

- Delay seeking appropriate treatments
- Undergo inappropriate treatments
- Waste precious healthcare dollars
- Adopt health regimens that, at best, do no good, and, at worst, do great harm

The suggestions for evaluation of health information that follow may seem like common sense (in fact, it is our hope that they are common sense), but they nonetheless can help healthcare consumers separate the scarce wheat from the all-too-abundant chaff of health information and avoid the harm caused by bad information.

135

Scientific Versus Nonscientific Medicine

To evaluate healthcare information, it is important to be aware of the differences between scientific and nonscientific medicine.

Scientific Medicine

Through the scientific method, scientists strive to create accurate representations of the world. All scientific investigation begins with a hypothesis followed by experimental tests that may either confirm or rule out the hypothesis. Most published scientific documents—especially journal articles—report the results of experiments. To be considered scientifically valid, experimental results must be reproducible by independent researchers. To keep the quality of the published scientific literature high, scientific documents often undergo peer review prior to publication. For those who embrace the principles of scientific medicine, no healthcare information is valid until its veracity has been proven through the application of the scientific method.

One of the staunchest proponents of scientific medicine—and a staunch opponent of nonscientific forms of alternative healthcare—is **Quackwatch** (*www.quackwatch.com*).

Nonscientific Medicine

Nonscientific medicine falls into two categories. First there is the type of medicine advocated by those who openly reject, to one extent or another, scientific medicine and the scientific method. For such advocates, applying the standards of scientific medicine to their approach to healthcare is as preposterous and offensive as evaluating one religion by the standards of another. Instead of following the scientific method, advocates of nonscientific medicine are guided by such factors as tradition, personal experience, religious beliefs, and other intangibles.

The second type of nonscientific medicine falls under the rubric of *pseudoscience*. Medicine of this sort dresses itself in the clothing of science but does not actually meet the standards imposed by the scientific method. You may be dealing with pseudoscientific information if it:

- Presents data based entirely on the findings of a single researcher or study
- Does not clearly identify studies to which it refers
- Makes grandiose claims for the effectiveness ("99.99% effective!") of a therapy

- Claims that a single therapy is effective for a large number of unrelated diseases or conditions
- Attacks all other therapies as useless or harmful
- Presents findings based on anecdotal information
- Does not acknowledge any limitations, areas of uncertainty, or potential risks
- Presents findings that have not—or cannot—be reproduced by independent researchers

With the growing acceptance of complementary and alternative medicine, there have been attempts to find common ground between scientific and nonscientific medicine. Notable among these attempts is the National Institutes of Health National Center for Complementary and Alternative Medicine (NCCAM). According to its promotional materials, "NCCAM is an advocate for quality science, rigorous and relevant research, and open and objective inquiry into which CAM [complementary and alternative medicine] practices work, which do not, and why."

You can visit the NCCAM Web site at *http://altmed.od.nih.gov.*

Who?

The most important question to ask when evaluating health information is, "Who is responsible for this information?"

THE FIRST RULE OF WHO

Whether the medium is online or print, those who publish health-related information should make it abundantly clear who they are. This rule holds true for individual as well as corporate authors, for informal as well as formal publications.[1] On many Web sites, information on who is responsible for the site and its content is found under an "About" link. Information that is presented anonymously should be considered unreliable until proven otherwise, as should information presented under a pseudonym.

WHO: QUALIFICATIONS

One way to evaluate health-related information is to consider the qualifications, including education and experience, of the authors of that information.

---

1. We are using the verb *to publish* in the broad sense of making a thing known. Under this definition, publications include everything from textbooks and peer-reviewed journals to personal Web pages and postings to electronic discussion groups.

Beware of those who try to hide their lack of qualifications under such hedges as "noted expert" or "prominent researcher" and then fail to state exactly when and where they have studied and worked. By the same token, do not be lulled into a false sense of security by those who would dazzle with the academic abbreviations that trail after their names. Bogus degrees obtained by mail order or made up out of whole cloth do not count as qualifications, nor does the fact that someone has a legitimate degree necessarily make that person an expert in every area of health care. An MD trained in neurology is not *de facto* an expert on nutrition. A researcher who holds a PhD in biochemistry may have less knowledge of asthma therapies than the checkout clerk at your local supermarket. (See "Evaluating Healthcare Professionals and Institutions" later in this chapter for detailed information on evaluating the education, skills, and experience of health professionals.)

WHO: AFFILIATION

Affiliation with prominent health-related government agencies, businesses, educational institutions, hospitals, nonprofit associations, research facilities, or scholarly/professional societies speaks well of an author's qualifications. If you suspect someone is being deceitful about an affiliation, you can surf the Web site of, or make a telephone call to, the alleged affiliated institution. Consulting the *Encyclopedia of Associations*[2] can help you verify the existence of—and determine the size, purpose, and prestige of—societies in which individuals claim membership.

Even when people have legitimate affiliations, it is worthwhile asking whether the information they are presenting is endorsed by the affiliated institution. For example, it is one thing for a member of the American Medical Association to present health-related information, but quite another for the AMA itself to put its imprimatur on that information. The same holds true of faculty members and the schools where they teach, of researchers and the facilities at which they work.

WHO: ORIGINAL CREATOR?

Especially in the Web environment, it is important to determine whether you are getting the information directly from the original creator or via someone else. In the latter case, you must ask if any changes—intentional or unintentional—have crept into the information.

Two cases, however, in which you need not much worry that the originator of the information was not personally responsible for putting the information online are electronic books and journals that are verbatim reproductions of print publications and official electronic publications of prominent businesses

---

2. Ballard, Patricia Tsune. *Encyclopedia of Associations: An Associations Unlimited Reference.* 37th ed. Detroit: Gale Research, 2001.

or organizations (for example, **MayoClinic.com** or **NIH Word on Health**). When dealing with such publications, you can rely on the editorial accuracy of the online publisher or aggregator to the same extent that you can rely on the editorial accuracy of a print publisher. This is not to say that significant changes between the original accepted manuscript and the final published item are impossible, but rather that they are uncommon.

Purpose

The purpose of health-related information generally falls under one or more of the following headings:

- Improve the quality of health (public or individual)
- Make a profit
- Enhance public relations
- Educate (consumers, healthcare professionals, or both)
- Promote a political, religious, or philosophical viewpoint
- Entertain

Of course it is possible for information to serve more than one purpose. Information provided by a pharmaceutical company may improve the quality of health while, at the same time, it may help the company both enhance its public image and increase its profits. Information intended to discourage teenagers from smoking may both educate and entertain.

It is important to note that there is nothing inherently wrong with any of the above purposes. In fact, it is hard to imagine information that does not have *some* purpose behind it. Alarms should go off, however, when the true purpose of information is obscured. Consider, for example, an organizational Web site (.org) devoted to a common childhood complaint. It champions a medical device as the best therapy for this complaint and, at the same time, the Web site stridently attacks the standard therapy, which employs medication. This Web site repeatedly offers visitors to the site the opportunity to purchase the medical device it promotes. Even though the Web site presents itself as a nonprofit, informational site, its main purpose seems to be to sell as many medical devices as possible. While it is not inappropriate to sell medical devices on the Web, it is difficult to trust the information provided by any Web site that pretends to serve one purpose while actually serving another.

The question of purpose leads directly to the problem of conflict of interest. A few typical examples of such conflict include:

- A Web site that accepts advertising refrains from presenting health information that could hurt a major advertiser's sales.
- A Web site that offers information on the benefits of vitamins provides

---

Print Versus Online Information

Both print and online health information must be evaluated. Something published in a respected, peer-reviewed journal or standard textbook of medicine is not automatically the final word on the subject, nor is something posted to an online discussion list automatically invalid. And, certainly, plenty of the health information published in mass-market print media is as bad as anything found on the Web.

---

links that allow readers to purchase these same vitamins online. The information provided by this Web site never mentions possible adverse effects of vitamins, nor is there any mention of the widely held opinion that vitamin supplements are unnecessary if one eats a healthy, balanced diet.

- A journal article based on research funded by the cattle industry comes out strongly in favor of a diet rich in red meat.
- A U.S. government health agency engages in self-censorship to avoid angering the chair of the Congressional committee that determines its funding.

Just as every piece of published information will have its purpose, it will also have its inevitable conflicts of interest. Healthcare consumers need to consider possible conflicts of interest and to weigh the effect of any such conflicts when evaluating healthcare information. Most important, consumers must cast a critical eye on sources of information that attempt to hide or gloss over conflicts of interest.

Currency

Because change is a constant in the world of health care, the currency of information is, in most cases, important to healthcare consumers. Any reliable source of information should tell you when it was first published (in print or electronically). If there was a significant lag time between creation and publication, the source should also indicate when the information was first created. When applicable, sources should give the date of the most recent update, and those sources updated on a regular basis should say how often they are updated (for example, daily, quarterly)

Audience

When evaluating healthcare information, consumers must consider the intended audience for that information. The two principal audiences for healthcare information are healthcare consumers and healthcare professionals (a broad group that may be categorized, for example, as medical doctors, PhDs, registered nurses, and physical therapists).

While it is possible that healthcare consumers might encounter information that is beneath their level (for example, the information might be intended for children), a more common problem is encountering highly technical information intended for healthcare professionals. For example, the *PubMed* database can point a healthcare consumer to abundant information on any medical topic, but that information is often too technical for all but medical experts. Medical dictionaries can help the average healthcare consumer interpret such information, but no dictionary is a substitute for a health professional's years of specialized education and experience. After all, how many lay persons know what to make of it when a journal article reports that a particular therapy has an NNT (Number Needed to Treat) of 15? Is that good or bad? Would a different therapy with an NNT of 10 be a better option? Compounding this problem is the fact that much of the information intended for healthcare professionals is not readily available to the average healthcare consumer. While the local public or college library will probably have subscriptions to *JAMA*, *Lancet*, and *New England Journal of Medicine*, only a good-sized medical library will have such titles as *Journal of Obstetrics and Gynaecology* or *European Journal of Surgical Oncology*.

Related to the topic of audience is the language of publication. Obviously, an English-language medical book will not be much help to someone who speaks only Spanish. For those serving communities of non-English-speaking healthcare consumers, finding information in the appropriate language can be a challenge.

Accuracy

Any information that is riddled with obvious errors (such as misspellings, grammatical errors, omitted words, or errors of fact) should be considered suspect. While it is true that the Web environment is more tolerant of misspellings and informal grammar than is the traditional print environment, accuracy still counts for something. Even a seemingly small error—such as typing "3cc" instead of "2cc"—could be dangerous when dealing with something as exact as pharmaceutical dosages.

Sources

Reliable sources of information accurately and completely cite the sources they consulted. Be especially leery of any source that throws around phrases like "studies show" without specifying exactly to what studies it is referring.

Independent Confirmation

If, for example, Source A claims that Drug X has shown promise as an allergy medication, it is good to find independent confirmation of that information before taking it as gospel. In general, the more sources agree on a point of fact or medical opinion (and the more varied those sources are), the more confidence you can have in that fact or opinion. Be sure, however, that the sources in agreement came to that consensus independently. On the Web, in particular, it is quite possible that all the various sources touting Drug X as an allergy medication got their information directly from Source A in the first place.

Reviews

Reviews can help consumers evaluate health-related books and Web sites. Reviews of health-related trade books can be found in mainstream review sources. The monthly magazine *Medicine on the Net* is an excellent source for print reviews of health-related Web sites.

Online reviews of print and electronic information are useful if you can locate them and if they are truly unbiased, independent reviews. Many online bookstores post customer-generated book reviews, which, if nothing else, give the popular reaction to a particular book. Typing the title of a health-related book into an Internet search engine will sometimes retrieve online reviews. Online reviews of Web sites can be difficult to find. It is common for Webmasters to make links to online reviews of their Web sites, but beware that such links almost never point to negative reviews and that some of the positive reviews may be neither unbiased nor independent of the source being reviewed.

Quality Control

Peer review, which is commonly used by scientific journals, requires that any manuscript must be approved by an impartial panel of experts prior to publication. While peer review can never be perfectly free of errors or bias, it represents the most rigorous quality control possible, and, for this reason, peer-reviewed publications are considered most reliable. Next on the quality-control scale are those publications in which a professional editor (or group of editors) decides what gets published and oversees quality control. With such publications, the knowledge, objectivity, and professionalism of the editor (or editors) is all-important to the quality of the final product, whether it appears in print or electronic form. On the Web just about anyone can set himself or herself up as an editor/publisher regardless of knowledge, objectivity, and professionalism (or complete lack thereof). In addition, for most electronic chat and discussion groups, there is no editorial (and so no quality) control whatsoever. All this adds up to the fact that the quality of information on the Web varies wildly.

Links

For Web sites that make large numbers of links to other Web sites, another aspect to consider is the criteria used when deciding what Web sites are worthy of a link. Comprehensive Web sites like **Yahoo!** (*www.yahoo.com*) make links to as many sites as possible without regard for the quality of those sites. On the other hand, selective Web sites like **healthfinder** (*www.healthfinder.gov*) and **NetWellness** (*www.netwellness.org*) require that the Web sites to which they link meet strict criteria.

As a general rule, good Web sites make good links; bad ones, bad links. Given this rule, one practical means for judging the quality of a health-related Web site is to look at the links it makes to other Web sites. A good Web site should:

- Link to other quality Web sites
- Link mostly or entirely to health-related Web sites rather than to Web sites covering unrelated topics
- Link to Web sites that represent more than one point of view
- Regularly review and update links, so that few or none point to Web sites that have either closed down or changed addresses
- Provide some information on how the linked Web sites are selected

Coverage

A source of consumer health information may be evaluated both by the information it includes and by what it excludes. The information included should be appropriate for the intended audience and purpose. A consumer health information source intended for children should not, for example, be loaded down with impenetrable scientific data culled from medical journals. Nor should a source that claims to be scientific in approach overload itself with nonscientific information.

Judging an information source by what it excludes is trickier than judging it by what it includes. How is the average person to know that a magazine article that cites three studies showing that Herbal Compound X is effective against hay fever has failed to cite the seven more recent studies showing Herbal Compound X to have no effect at all? The answer is that, without some research, there is no way to know this. Still, it helps to be alert for major gaps in coverage. For example, it would be difficult to trust an information source that purports to list every breast cancer therapy if that source then fails to include chemotherapy on the list.

Usability

Good organization, indexes, tables of contents, clear layout, informative illustrations, and readable type all contribute to the usability of print information sources. Similarly, for a Web site to be usable, the information it contains needs to be organized so that users can find what they are looking for quickly and easily. The Web site's most important information should be featured on the homepage and be accessible with only a click or two. Site indexes, internal search engines, navigation bars, and logically organized subject categories can also help to guide visitors through a Web site. The graphic design of a Web site should contribute to usability; the design should provide a consistent look but not be so extravagant as to interfere with navigation. It is also important to remember that cool graphics, sharp layout, and flashy special effects do not mean that the information provided by a Web site is good information. It is relatively easy to make a Web site look cool, but relatively difficult to fill it with quality information.

Disclaimers and Privacy

Sources of consumer health information should provide disclaimers that acknowledge the limitations of such information. In particular, disclaimers should say that information (whether print or electronic) is not a substitute for a professional medical opinion.

If a consumer health Web site collects *any* information about you, it should have an easy-to-find privacy policy that tells you exactly what is and is not done with that information. Ideally, the Web site should also allow you to see all information it has collected about you and to make changes to, or deletions from, that information. Unless you give your consent, no Web site should share private information about you with partners, advertisers, or other third parties. Be aware that even Web sites with privacy policies have been known to violate those policies and that once you click a link and leave a Web site, its privacy policy no longer applies.

Privacy can be a concern with noncommercial as well as commercial Web sites. For example, the Web site of a major national, nonprofit disease association has an online grocery-store tour designed to teach those who suffer from the disease how to buy wisely. To take the tour, a visitor must first complete an extensive questionnaire (providing name, address, and phone number), yet there is nothing on the Web site that says what may, or may not, be done with this information. To cast even more suspicion, the online tour is sponsored by companies that manufacture foods frequently purchased by those who suffer from the disease in question.

Awards

The fact that an author, print publication, or Web site has won awards may testify to the credibility of the information presented, but such awards are not an absolute guarantee of quality. For one famous example, Dr. Linus Pauling's work in chemistry helped shape the face of scientific medicine, yet despite his two Nobel prizes, his theories on vitamin C and nutrition therapy remain highly controversial within the scientific community.

On the Web, many Web sites sport icons declaring that they are award-winning sites. Most of these icons, and the awards they represent, are meaningless. An exception is the HONcode icon. Created by the nonprofit Health on the Net Foundation, the HONcode icon is neither an award nor a rating of the quality of the information provided by the Web site. Instead, sites that display the HONcode icon have agreed to adhere to a set of ethical standards developed by the HON Foundation. For more information, visit the HON Foundation Web site at *www.hon.ch*.

The Mutability of Health Information

A common complaint about health information goes something like this: "One day some expert is telling you to eat oat bran, then the next day another expert is telling you 'Don't bother.' You might as well eat whatever you want because nobody really knows." Such fatalism is understandable in a culture where we are bombarded with conflicting information about what is and is not healthy, but those who tune out health information altogether are missing a few vital points:

- Scientific findings change because it is the nature of science to experiment continually, make new discoveries, and change the way we look at the world. When science becomes immutable, it is no longer science.
- Part of the appeal of many alternative therapies is that, unlike therapies based on scientific health care, they remain constant. While the timeless quality of such therapies may be a source of assurance, it is important to remember that therapies that never change also never improve.
- Science, though extremely objective when carried out according to its own rules, is nonetheless a human activity and, therefore, never perfect. Though to a lesser degree than in any other human endeavor, error, emotion, and desire can all interfere with scientific objectivity.

What happens, however, when despite a consumer's best effort to seek out the final word on a health-related topic, it ends up that equally reliable sources of information come to different conclusions? What does a consumer do, for example, when the science-oriented Center for Science in the Public Interest (*www.cspinet.org*) makes a convincing argument against the fat substitute Olestra while the science-oriented *American Council on Science and Health* (*www.acsh.org*) makes an equally convincing argument that Olestra is safe? The answer is that information can take us only so far. It can help us make better, more informed decisions about our health, but it cannot make deci-

---

Web Sources for Evaluating Health Information

Criteria for Assessing the Quality of Health Information on the Internet—Policy Paper
http://hitiweb.mitretek.org/docs/criteria.html
> Authored by the Health Information Technology Institute of Mitretek Systems, a nonprofit systems engineering company, this policy paper spells out specific criteria for evaluating health information.

DISCERN Instrument
www.discern.org.uk/discern_instrument.htm
> The *DISCERN Instrument* consists of a series of questions designed to help users rate sources of consumer health information. The DISCERN project is based in the University of Oxford Division of Public Health and Primary Health Care at the Institute of Health Sciences.

Tips on Evaluating Web Resources
www.nnlm.nlm.nih.gov/gmr/publish/eval.html
> A quick and handy tip sheet produced by the National Network of Libraries of Medicine Greater Midwest Region.

Tip-Offs to Rip-Offs
www.arthritis.org/alttherapies/default.asp#tip
> Helpful evaluation pointers from the Arthritis Foundation and a good example of the type of publication that could be distributed directly to healthcare consumers.

---

sions for us. In the end, it is up to each of us to decide how we will care for our own health.

Evaluating Healthcare Professionals and Institutions

The most common way for consumers to evaluate healthcare professionals is through word of mouth. A doctor's former patients—whether they are friends of the consumer, family members, or strangers—can all provide valuable word-of-mouth recommendations. However, perhaps before trusting life and limb to a complete stranger in a white coat, a healthcare consumer might want to know a bit more than, "When my brother George got cancer, Doctor X was just so caring and kind. He even came to the funeral." The sources and approaches discussed in this section can help consumers find the best information on which to base decisions concerning who will care for them and where.

Evaluating Doctors

"How good is Doctor X?" is a common question for healthcare consumers. This question might be asked about a specialist on whose skills and knowledge a life depends, or it might be asked about a primary care physician who is with the consumer's HMO. In either case, it is not a simple question to answer.

EDUCATION AND EXPERIENCE

Two important standards by which doctors are measured are their education and experience. Questions to consider when it comes to a doctor's education include:

- Where and when did the doctor go to medical school?
  — Was it an accredited medical school?
- Where and when did the doctor do his or her residency?
  — Was it an accredited residency?
  — What specialty was the residency in?
- Did the doctor participate in a fellowship after residency?
- How long has the doctor been practicing medicine?

Very often you can find the answers to the above questions by consulting any or all of the following sources:

AMA Physician Select
www.ama-assn.org/aps/amahg.htm

Directory of Physicians in the United States[3]

HealthGrades.com
www.healthgrades.com

DoctorDirectory.com
www.doctordirectory.com

For more specific questions—such as "How many times has Dr. X performed this operation he wants to do on me?"—the consumer has little recourse other than to ask Dr. X for the information.

PROFESSIONAL ASSOCIATION MEMBERSHIPS

Finding out what professional associations a physician belongs to can tell you something about the physician's interests and his or her involvement in the

---

3. *Directory of Physicians in the United States.* Chicago: American Medical Association, 1992–.

profession. For example, a consumer might choose a pediatrician who is a member of the American Academy of Pediatrics over one who is not. The best way to find out what professional associations a physician belongs to is to ask the physician directly. As mentioned above, most questions about the size and significance of a professional association can be answered by the *Encyclopedia of Associations*. A visit to a specific association's Web site can also be informative.

LICENSURE

Licensed physicians (both medical doctors and doctors of osteopathy) have the legal right to diagnose and treat patients without supervision. Each state has its own medical licensing board for physicians, and requirements for licensure vary from state to state. In general, an individual must have a certain level of education and pass an examination in order to be licensed as a physician. Many states also require that physicians take a certain amount of continuing medical education (CME) in order to keep their medical licenses current. The surest way to find out if a particular doctor has a current license is to check with the appropriate state medical board. The Federation of State Medical Boards (FSMB) maintains a directory of state medical boards at *www.fsmb.org/members.htm*. You can get information on the role and function of state medical boards from the FSMB homepage at *www.fsmb.org*.

BOARD CERTIFICATION

While a license is required in order to practice medicine, board certification is optional; in theory, any licensed physician can work in any specialty or subspecialty without being board certified, though the reality of malpractice insurance will usually prevent, say, an orthopedic surgeon from casually setting up shop as a psychiatrist. Board certification is not absolutely required because it is granted not by governmental agencies, but rather by professional societies representing the various medical specialties. To be board certified, physicians must have a specific level of education (a medical degree plus a three- to seven-year residency), pass an intensive written examination in their specialty or subspecialty, and possibly meet other requirements. In some specialties, physicians must take continuing medical education and/or periodically retake the certification examination to remain board certified. To find out if a physician is board certified, consult one of the following sources:

> *The Official ABMS Directory of Board Certified Medical Specialists*[4] (a multivolume set published annually by the American Board of Medical Specialties)
> "Who's Certified," a section of the ABMS Web site (*www.abms.org*)

---

4. *The Official ABMS Directory of Board Certified Medical Specialists, 2001.* 33rd ed. New Providence, N.J.: Marquis Who's Who, 2001.

While board certification is one important criterion for measuring the knowledge and skill of a physician, it is important to remember that there are bad doctors who are board certified just as there are good doctors who are not.

DISCIPLINARY ACTION

"Has Doctor X ever been disciplined?" can be a hard question to answer because information about disciplinary action is often unavailable or buried so deep that it is difficult to find. Compounding the problem is the fact that U.S. physicians can be disciplined not only by their state medical boards, but also by the Drug Enforcement Administration (for over-prescribing certain controlled drugs), the Department of Health and Human Services (for Medicare or Medicaid fraud), and the Food and Drug Administration (for violating rules covering clinical research on patients).

As with questions about licensure, the place to start with questions about disciplinary action is with the appropriate state medical board. State medical boards can discipline doctors for a number of reasons, some of them of great concern to patients (incompetence, negligence, substance abuse), others, of almost no concern (failing to repay student loans). Sanctions can range from mandatory remedial education to reprimands to permanent loss of license. The amount of disciplinary information state medical boards provide to the public varies from state to state. Residents of Maine, for example, can go to the Maine Board of Medical Licensure Web site (*www.docboard.org/me/ me_home.htm*) to see a detailed list of "Adverse Licensing Actions" taken by the board. Residents of other states may need to dig deeper. The Federation of State Medical Boards directory (*www.fsmb.org/members.htm*) is a good starting point to find out what disciplinary information is available in a particular state.

The multivolume *Questionable Doctors Disciplined by State and Federal Governments*[5] provides detailed information on disciplinary actions taken against specific doctors. Published at irregular intervals by Public Citizen Health Research Group (a nonprofit watchdog group founded by Ralph Nader), it covers various states or regions of the country.

Another avenue for finding out if a physician has been sanctioned is the *Sanction Search* feature at *www.doctordirectory.com*. For a fee ($9.95 in fall 2000), *Sanction Search* will provide a report detailing any sanctions on the license of a specific doctor.

A final note about disciplinary action: For the most part, state medical boards wait until patients complain before investigating physicians. This means that physicians who are entirely deserving of discipline might have clean records simply because none of their patients ever complained about them.

---

5. Wolfe, Sidney M. "Questionable Doctors Disciplined by State and Federal Governments." Washington, D.C.: Public Citizen's Health Research Group, 2000.

MALPRACTICE

When medical boards discipline physicians, they follow formal processes of complaint and investigation, observing due process and holding hearings. So, as a rule, a disciplinary action indicates that some real violation has actually taken place. On the other hand, anyone can bring a malpractice suit whether there are grounds for the suit or not. Just because a physician (or any other healthcare provider) has been sued does not necessarily mean that wrong was done. Even in a malpractice suit in which a settlement is paid out to a plaintiff, it may be the case that the doctor did no wrong—insurance companies often decide to settle purely for economic reasons, regardless of the physician's guilt or innocence.

If a number of malpractice suits have been brought against a physician, this may indicate a pattern of incompetence or negligence. However, finding out if a physician has been sued, and how often, is not always easy. Some state medical boards provide information about suits brought against physicians; however, it may be necessary to undertake a potentially costly search of court records to determine if, or how often, a particular doctor has been sued.

Evaluating Other Healthcare Professionals

Most of the factors used to evaluate physicians can also be used to evaluate other healthcare professionals (dentists, nurses, physical therapists, psychologists, alternative healers, and so on). As with a physician, you can start by checking out a healthcare professional's education and experience, but unlike physicians, there may be no central directory that gives this information for the type of healthcare professional you are evaluating. The best solution for the healthcare consumer may be to ask the healthcare professional directly about his or her education and experience.

LICENSURE, DISCIPLINARY ACTIONS, AND MALPRACTICE

If the healthcare professional you are evaluating is a member of a licensed profession, then the state board that licenses that profession is the first place to turn to for information about licensure, disciplinary action, or malpractice suits. In some states, the same medical board that licenses physicians also licenses other health professions; in other states, there may be separate boards for psychologists, nurses, and so on. For questions about licensure, disciplinary actions, or malpractice involving non-physician healthcare professionals, try the following Web sites:

Federation of Chiropractic Licensing Boards
www.fclb.org
American Association of Dental Examiners
www.aadexam.org

Two Useful Sources for Finding Good Doctors

Best Doctors
www.bestdoctors.com

Best Doctors is a fee-based service designed to help healthcare consumers locate the best doctors by medical specialty and location. *Best Doctors* conducts nationwide surveys of doctors to find out which doctors are most recommended by their peers. Only board-certified doctors are included in *Best Doctors*, and doctors who have been sanctioned by state medical boards are excluded. According to its own promotional materials, *Best Doctors* is "completely independent. Doctors are not asked for and do not ever pay any fees for inclusion as a Best Doctor."

Guide to Top Doctors[6]

Guide to Top Doctors lists some 15,000 top-rated physicians in 50 major metropolitan areas. Physicians' ratings are based on surveys of physicians, and each entry includes information on the physician's training, credentials and office locations. The publishers of *Guide to Top Doctors* do not accept advertising and prohibit the use of their publications for commercial purposes, including advertising.

National Council of Boards of Nursing
www.ncsbn.org/files/boards.asp
National Board for Certification in Occupational Therapy
www.nbcot.org
Member Boards
www.iabopt.org/about/MemberBoards.asp
Directory of State Boards
www.fsbpt.org/directory.cfm
Physician Assistant State Regulatory Agencies
www.aapa.org/gandp/statereg.html
Association of State and Provincial Psychology Boards
www.asppb.org
State Agencies for Licensure [respiratory therapists]
www.nbrc.org/agencies.htm

Not every health profession falls into a neat category. For example, nurse midwives are licensed by boards of nursing in some states, by boards of medi-

---

6. *Guide to Top Doctors*. Washington, D.C.: Center for the Study of Services, 1999.

cine in others. When looking for licensure, disciplinary, or malpractice information about a healthcare profession not listed above, try locating the homepage of the national association for the profession in question. A good place to begin a search for such association homepages is **MedWeb** at *www.MedWeb.Emory.Edu/MedWeb*. Once at the **MedWeb** site, look in the "Institutions" category and then find the link to "Societies."[7]

NONLICENSED HEALTHCARE PRACTITIONERS

It is very difficult to evaluate healthcare practitioners in fields that are not licensed, which is the case with many forms of alternative health care. Just about anyone could, for example, go into business as an aromatherapist or a gemstone therapist—no license, education, or clear idea of what one is doing is required. It is possible to check the educational credentials of practitioners in unregulated fields of health care, but because many schools that teach this type of health care are unaccredited, it can be hard to tell if a practitioner's educational credentials are worth any more than the paper on which they are printed.

Other than word of mouth, perhaps the best way for a healthcare consumer to evaluate a practitioner in an unregulated field is to learn as much as possible about that field and make an evaluation based on the practitioner's apparent knowledge or lack thereof.

Evaluating Hospitals

When it comes to getting basic facts about virtually any hospital in the United States, the bible is the *AHA Guide to the Health Care Field.*[8] The *AHA Guide* provides such data as number of beds, number of employees, kinds of services offered, and so on. Similar data can be found by clicking on the "Free Services" link found on the **American Hospital Directory** (*www.ahd.com*). Two other notable Web resources for evaluating hospitals are:

Best Hospitals Finder
  www.usnews.com/usnews/nycu/health/hosptl/tophosp.htm
  Best Hospitals Finder, a product of *U.S. News & World Report*, ranks hospitals in 17 specialty areas. Rankings are based on reputation, mortality rates, and other factors.

---

7. The direct URL to MedWeb's "Societies" link is quite convoluted: *www.MedWeb.Emory. Edu/MedWeb/FMPro?-DB=secondaries.FP3&-Format=Secondary.htm&-Lay=Web&-Max=1000&-Op=eq&Index==Societies_and_Associations:*&-Sortfield=Sec&-Token=Societies_and_Associations:&-Find.*

8. *AHA Guide to the Health Care Field.* Chicago: Healthcare Infosource, 1997–.

HealthGrades
www.healthgrades.com
HealthGrades employs a complex statistical methodology to rate hospitals, physicians, health plans, nursing homes, home health agencies, hospice programs, and fertility clinics. Explanations of the **HealthGrades** methodologies are available on the Web site. **HealthGrades** is a for-profit business. It accepts advertising and licenses the commercial use of its name, data, and ratings by those individuals and institutions that it rates.

Teach Healthcare Consumers to Evaluate for Themselves

Anyone who teaches (or shows) healthcare consumers how to find information should also teach them how to evaluate it. In an informal situation, such teaching might take the form of a quick reminder that "There's a lot of bad information out there. Don't trust everything you read," or "You can find all kinds of information about arthritis, but the sources that I trust the most are . . . ." In more formal classroom settings, evaluation should be stressed again and again. One of the best ways to make learners aware of the need to evaluate is to demonstrate a few extremely wacky sources of health information—examples are appallingly easy to find on the Web. Teachers should also give learners tips on how to evaluate. Handouts with titles like "Red Flags for Fraudulent Healthcare Information" or "Six Questions to Ask When Evaluating Healthcare Information" can be useful in the classroom as well as at the reference desk. How you communicate the evaluation message is less important than the fact that the message be an integral part of your efforts to put consumers in touch with healthcare information.

9
Creating Effective Print Consumer Health Publications for Your Users

A consumer health publication can take many forms, including:

- **Bibliography.** This might consist of a list of health-related books, Web sites, or journal articles. Adding annotations helps consumers judge the usefulness of the resources listed.
- **Referral.** This type of publication provides contact information for anything from local clinics to national disease associations to online support groups. Along with physical addresses and telephone numbers, referral publications usually provide Web addresses (URLs) and e-mail addresses.
- **How-to information.** Such a publication tells consumers the best way to do something, whether it be searching a medical database, researching a specific disease or condition, or evaluating healthcare information.
- **Basic health facts.** A publication of this type generally focuses on a specific disease or condition and includes information on causes, symptoms, and therapies.

Whether a consumer health publication takes on one of the forms described above, a combination of these forms, or some other form altogether, the overall success of a publication depends on three things: writing, layout, and distribution.

Writing a Consumer Health Publication

Is There a Need?

Before taking on the job of writing, laying out, and distributing a consumer health publication, the first question to ask is, "Is there a need for this publication?" Consumer demand for information on a particular health topic may make the need for a relevant publication seem obvious, but even in the face of high demand it is worth investigating the true extent of the need. For example, there might be a sudden, heavy demand for information on migraines because of a *Sixty Minutes* segment on the topic; this demand, however, may prove to be short-lived and a publication on the topic not worth the bother. On the other hand, questions about childhood immunizations may be perennial and, thus, well served by a publication. Talking to librarians, healthcare professionals, and healthcare consumers is the best way to get a sense of whether an apparent need for a consumer health publication is genuine.

A second important question is whether there already is a good consumer health publication on your proposed topic. If your proposed topic is local in focus—for example, a bibliography of diabetes information resources available in your library or a directory of local clinics that provide childhood immunizations—then it is unlikely that a similar publication already exists. On the other hand, if the topic of your proposed publication concerns a major disease, condition, or a matter of general public health and safety, it is likely that a health-related association, society, or government agency already makes available relevant consumer health publications that can be either reproduced and distributed without copyright restrictions or purchased in bulk for less than the cost of developing and printing similar documents in house. For just one of many examples, the Centers for Disease Control and Prevention offers a free publication (in both English and Spanish) on preventing Hantavirus; like most government publications, it can be downloaded via the Web (*www.cdc.gov/ncidod/diseases/hanta/hps/noframes/prevcard.htm*) and freely reproduced without any copyright restriction. By taking advantage of existing free or low-cost consumer health publications, you not only save yourself the expense and trouble of creating a new publication, you also avoid any liability as creator of such a publication.

When looking for existing consumer health publications, a good starting point is the National Library of Medicine's **MEDLINE***plus* (*www.medlineplus.gov*). Other good sources for free or low-cost publications are health-related associations and societies, such as the American Cancer Society, the American Academy of Pediatrics, the Muscular Dystrophy Association, and so on. For a list of health-related associations and societies on the Web, see the "Associations" page on Emory University's **MedWeb** (*www.medweb.emory.edu*).

Of course before you reproduce and distribute numerous copies of any existing consumer health publication, you will want to check directly with the publication's creator/copyright holder to verify that the publication is freely available for duplication. To be completely safe, obtain the creator/copyright holder's written permission to copy and distribute. Even if the publication is free, the person, agency, or association that created the publication will most often want you to give proper credit on all copies you distribute.

Purpose and Audience

Once you have determined that there is a need for a consumer health publication on a particular topic, you must ask yourself, "What is the purpose of this publication?" Is it to help consumers use health resources in the public library? Help senior citizens find and evaluate health information on the Web? Make low-income mothers aware of services offered by local well-baby clinics? Inform the public about a disease or condition? Save reference librarians the work of answering a consumer health question that gets asked 20 times a day? Whatever it may be, the purpose of a publication should be your polestar throughout the development process. Anything that leads away from the purpose has no place in the publication.

Equally important to purpose is the publication's audience. Ask yourself, "Who am I writing this for?" Librarians? Health professionals? Social workers? Senior citizens? Parents? Children? Always think about your audience and try to think like them. Try to anticipate anything that might be a stumbling block to your audience:

- Is illiteracy a problem?
- Would diagrams be more effective than words with this audience?
- Are there cultural issues to be aware of to avoid offending audience members?
- Does the typeface need to be large so that older eyes can read it clearly?
- Should this publication be produced in other languages besides English?

Whoever your audience may be, piloting a draft of your publication with multiple members of that audience is an excellent strategy:

- Does the pilot audience find the level of the writing so high as to be incomprehensible, or so low as to be insulting?
- Do the images used in the publication send a message you did not intend?
- Do native speakers of the publication's language identify any problems?
- Would the pilot audience prefer that the publication serve a different purpose than the one you chose?
- Would the pilot audience prefer that the publication address another topic altogether?
- Are any parts of the publication confusing to the pilot audience?

Content

Of course any self-respecting consumer health publication should provide valid, accurate content. For bibliographic and referral publications, basic facts (such as URLs, call numbers, citations, addresses, and phone numbers) must be impeccably accurate. Such accuracy demands tedious, but absolutely necessary, checking and rechecking. (**Tip:** When including URLs in a publication, accuracy is best served by copying URLs directly from the Web page in question and pasting them into the publication. Typing URLs inevitably leads to errors.)

For publications that contain basic health facts (for example, the causes, symptoms, and standard treatments for hepatitis C), you should consult a number of standard information sources and summarize their findings. You might also do well to engage the services of one or more licensed health professionals who are willing to review the accuracy and validity of any such publications. (See sidebar: "Over the Line?")

Once the content of a publication has been tested on a pilot audience, it is necessary to proofread the publication carefully for grammar errors, spelling errors, and other mistakes. Having different people proofread a publication is essential, as a single proofreader can easily pass over the same error more than once without noticing it. Getting a pair of "fresh eyes" (someone who has never before seen the publication) to proofread during the final stages of production is an excellent strategy. Remember that once you have sent a publication to the print shop or run off a few hundred copies on the office photocopier, all the regret in the world will not correct a misspelling or convert the "3" in that crucial phone number into the "5" it was *supposed* to have been. Proofread, proofread, proofread.

Finally, do not forget the following:

- **Date consumer health publications.** A prominent date not only alerts the public to the possibility that the information may be out of date, but it also serves to remind you when it is time to update a publication.
- **Identify your institution.** Anyone who reads your publication should know what library, association, or agency produced it. This information not only helps the reader evaluate the content of the publication, but also raises awareness of your institution.
- **Provide contact information.** Readers should know how to contact your institution for more information. Contact information should include physical address, phone number (with area code), e-mail contact address, and Web site address (URL). Yes, even if a publication is entirely Web-based, include a physical address and phone number. If someone on the staff is the designated consumer health contact, his or her name can be part of the contact information as well.

Organization

A logically organized publication will more effectively serve its purpose than one that has been thrown together haphazardly. This section describes a number of effective organizational schemes for consumer health publications.

QUESTION AND ANSWER

Stating common questions and following each with an answer is a good way to organize almost any short publication such as a brochure or flyer. On the

Over the Line?

Unless you are a licensed health professional, you do not want to put yourself into the position of dispensing medical advice. This means you must not create consumer health publications that diagnose or prescribe therapies for diseases and conditions. It is acceptable to list generally accepted symptoms, causes, and therapies, but if you do so, it is important to include a disclaimer that says something to the effect that:

1. The information provided in this publication is not intended as informed medical advice.
2. No one should attempt to diagnose or treat a condition or disease without consulting a qualified healthcare provider.

Perusing the disclaimers found on most print and Web-based consumer health publications will give you plenty of ideas for writing your own disclaimer.

Another way to protect yourself from going too far in a consumer health publication is to cite a specific source for anything that might be considered a diagnosis or therapy. For example, you are pretty safe writing something like:

> *Griffith's 5-Minute Clinical Consult* (1999) lists symptoms of heat stroke as exhaustion; confusion or disorientation; coma; hot, flushed, dry skin; and a core temperature over 105° F.

Another strategy for protecting yourself and your organization is to find a qualified, licensed healthcare professional who is willing to author the publication or coauthor it with you. This way, at the very least, you cannot be accused of dispensing medical advice without a license.

Finally, if you are genuinely concerned over whether the content of a consumer health publication crosses the line between providing information and supplying medical advice, the best course is to seek guidance from one or more experts in law and medicine and to revise according to their advice.

Web, documents organized in this way are called FAQs (Frequently Asked Questions), and computer-literate audiences will be especially comfortable with this format. It is worthwhile to pilot question-and-answer documents with potential audience members, as this process will help you know if you have asked the right questions and answered them clearly. As far as layout goes, formatting questions differently from answers helps make question-and-answer publications easier to follow. For example, you might format the ques-

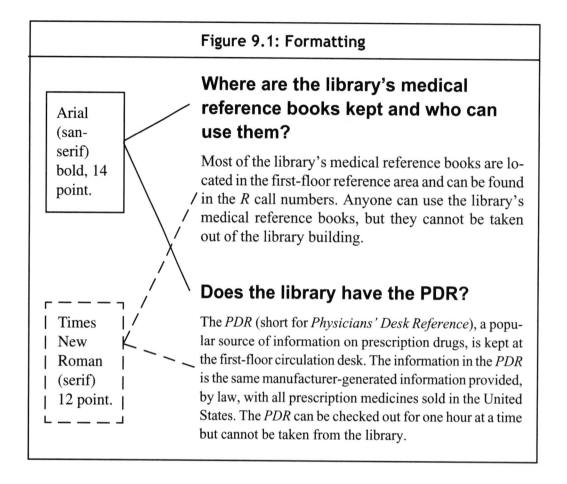

Figure 9.1: Formatting

Arial (san-serif) bold, 14 point.

Times New Roman (serif) 12 point.

Where are the library's medical reference books kept and who can use them?

Most of the library's medical reference books are located in the first-floor reference area and can be found in the *R* call numbers. Anyone can use the library's medical reference books, but they cannot be taken out of the library building.

Does the library have the PDR?

The *PDR* (short for *Physicians' Desk Reference*), a popular source of information on prescription drugs, is kept at the first-floor circulation desk. The information in the *PDR* is the same manufacturer-generated information provided, by law, with all prescription medicines sold in the United States. The *PDR* can be checked out for one hour at a time but cannot be taken from the library.

tions in a bold, sans-serif font and the answers in an unbolded serif font. If you are using spot color, printing the question in the spot color and the answers in black is an effective technique (see Figure 9.1).

Chronological

Much like a well-written cookbook recipe, publications organized chronologically take a "First this, then this, then this" approach. An effective organizational scheme for describing any linear (or nearly linear) process that involves steps, chronological organization lends itself well to how-to instructions. Consider Figure 9.2.

General to Specific

General to specific is yet another good way to organize guides to the literature on a consumer health topic. For example, a guide to consumer health information on diabetes might start by listing general medical references such as *Dorland's Illustrated Medical Dictionary* or *The New Wellness Encyclopedia* and then work toward more diabetes-specific sources, such as the book *Dia-*

Figure 9.2: Chronological Organization

How to Access MEDLINEplus from Public Computers in the Killdare Medical Library:

1. Click on the Netscape icon and wait for the Kildare Library homepage to load.
2. Click on the words **Health Information Links** (look in the column on the left-hand side of the screen).
3. Click on words **MEDLINEplus** (look near the top of the screen).

---

betes A to Z[1] or a specific page on the American Diabetes Association's Web site.

CAUSES, SYMPTOMS, AND TREATMENTS

Causes, symptoms, and treatments is a common method of organization for publications dealing with a specific disease or condition. Be aware that a publication organized in this way can easily cross the line into the realm of dispensing medical advice.

ORDER OF IMPORTANCE

Order of importance (either least-to-most or most-to-least) can be used to organize anything from a list of alternative medicine books to a brochure covering steps for keeping *E. coli* out of the home kitchen.

LIST OF DO'S AND DON'TS

This format lends itself well to a two-column layout with **Do's** in one column and **Don'ts** in the other. Be careful with this format, as it is surprisingly easy to put a **Do** in the **Don't** column and vice-versa.

CHECKLIST

Checklists are great for describing anything that involves a large number of steps or has many facets. Checklists are often organized chronologically or by order of importance (see Figure 9.3).

LOCATION

Organization by location is effective when the purpose is to tell people where to find something. A brochure listing free health clinics in your county might

---

1. Amercan Diabetes Association. *Diabetes A to Z: What You Need to Know About Diabetes, Simply Put, 4th Ed.* Alexandria, VA: American Diabetes Association, 2000.

Figure 9.3: Checklists

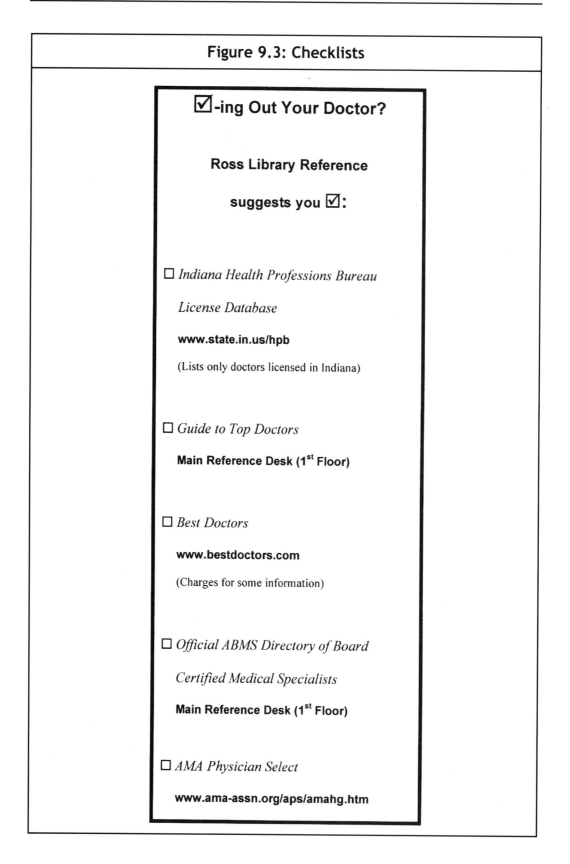

☑-ing Out Your Doctor?

Ross Library Reference

suggests you ☑:

☐ *Indiana Health Professions Bureau*

License Database

www.state.in.us/hpb

(Lists only doctors licensed in Indiana)

☐ *Guide to Top Doctors*

Main Reference Desk (1ˢᵗ Floor)

☐ *Best Doctors*

www.bestdoctors.com

(Charges for some information)

☐ *Official ABMS Directory of Board*

Certified Medical Specialists

Main Reference Desk (1ˢᵗ Floor)

☐ *AMA Physician Select*

www.ama-assn.org/aps/amahg.htm

be organized by the cities in which the clinics are located. A guide to a library's consumer health resources might group the resources by their location in the library: Reference Area, Reserve Desk, Books Stacks, Computer Cluster.

COMBINATIONS OF THE ABOVE

It is common to use combinations of the above methods of organization in a single publication. For example, a checklist or a list of Do's and Don'ts might be a section of a longer publication.

Laying Out a Consumer Health Publication

Before setting out to develop a consumer health publication, it is a good idea to look at lots of other publications—flyers, booklets, brochures, and so on. The publications need not be health related because you are looking at them with an eye for their appearance, not their content. Ask yourself questions about the publications you come across:

- What is the first thing I notice about the publication?
- What do I like about it?
- What do I dislike?
- How effectively does the publication use images?
- How effectively does the publication use typefaces?
- How effectively does the publication use white space?
- How does the layout of the publication emphasize (or fail to emphasize) its most important points?
- Is it easy or hard to follow the flow of the main points as I scan the publication?
- Does the layout serve the purpose of the publication well?

General Format

After you have decided what information will go into a publication, the next big decision will be the overall format of the publication. Will it be a single sheet of paper printed front and back? A bi-fold or tri-fold brochure? A side-stapled or saddle-stitched booklet? A specialty format such as a bookmark, recipe card, oversized matchbook, or comic book? The choice of format will depend on your audience, the type and quantity of information you intend to include, and your budget. Obviously, a standard format (such as an 8.5-by–11-inch flyer) that can be run off on an in-house photocopier is going to be less costly than a specialty format.

```
┌──────────────────────────────────────────────────────────┐
│           Figure 9.4: Serif and Sans Serif Typefaces      │
├──────────────────────────────────────────────────────────┤
│                                                            │
│  Serif typefaces have short lines (serifs) extending from  │
│  the upper and lower ends of the strokes of each letter.   │
│  Serif typefaces are often used for body text. Times New   │
│  Roman is a very common serif typeface.                    │
│                                                            │
│  The strokes of sans-serif (without serif) letters have    │
│  no lines extending from them. Sans-serif typefaces are    │
│  sometimes used for titles and headings. Arial is a        │
│  common sans-serif typeface.                               │
│                                                            │
└──────────────────────────────────────────────────────────┘
```

Emphasis

Boldface, color, italics, underlining, bullets, and shading can all be used to add emphasis within a publication. The trick to emphasis is not to overuse it. If you make every word in a publication bold, for example, the effect is lost and nothing stands out.

White Space

A common mistake is to try to crowd too much into a publication. Too much text (gray space) makes a publication look forbidding, like something difficult to read and comprehend. Too many images make a publication busy and hard to follow. As important as what you have to say and show might be, you must incorporate enough white space—margins, space around images, space between blocks of text—to give the eye a place to rest. White space also allows important points to stand out instead of being buried in a flood of text and images.

Typefaces

The two main kinds of typefaces are serif and sans serif, as shown in Figure 9.4.

The most important thing about typefaces is to choose a readable one for the body text of any publication. Fancy typefaces like Algerian or Mistral may be eye-catching, but in anything more than small doses they are eye-straining. Unless you purposely want a typewriter effect, use a proportionally spaced typeface, not a fixed-width typeface such as Courier. The second most important thing about typefaces is not to use too many typefaces in a single publication. More than two typefaces in a single short publication is probably too many. If you need typographical variety, try using different sizes and weights (boldface, lightface) of the same typeface.

Figure 9.5: Point Size for Typefaces

This is 10-point Times New Roman.

This is 10-point Arial.

This is 10-point Garamond.

For body text, choose a size of type (point size) that is big enough to be easily read. While the readability of print varies from typeface to typeface, 10-point type is about as small as you want to go. If a number of seniors will be using a publication, you may want to use an even larger type.

Alignment

In most cases, use left-aligned text with a ragged right-hand margin. Other options for alignment appear in Figure 9.6.

Color

Color can add to a publication's eye appeal and can also be used to emphasize important points. Full-color publications (called four-color in the printing trade)

Figure 9.6: Alignment of Text

Centering
is fine for titles and major headings.
But more than two or three consecutive lines
of centered text becomes hard to read.

Right-aligned text is even more difficult to read than centered text and is
almost never used with European languages.

Justified text, in which both left- and right-hand margins are flush, can look good if properly done, but justified text appears amateurish if words end up spaced too far apart or if lakes and rivers of white space flow through the paragraphs.

---

are attractive, but commercial printers will charge a premium for four-color printing, and in-house printing on a color printer or color photocopier will quickly eat up expensive color toner cartridges.

A cost-effective and attractive option to four-color printing is spot printing. With spot printing, you use one color of ink (usually black) for the main text and a second color of ink (the spot color) for emphasis. For example, you might use the spot color for headlines, bullets, and decorative lines. The trick is not to use the second color so much that emphasis is lost in a flood of color. Though less costly than four-color printing, spot printing is still more expensive than using a single ink color.

If color printing of any sort is a budget buster, it is still possible to enhance publications by printing black ink on colored paper. When choosing paper colors, make sure that there is good contrast between the color of the paper and the color of the ink. Super-bright paper colors are eye-catching but border on the painful when used for publications that require more than a quick glance.

Paper

Besides color, paper choices include weight, texture, and size. Twenty-pound bond, the standard for photocopier paper, is acceptable for most publications. Heavier weight paper, glossy paper, textured paper, or paper with high cotton content all make for a more impressive look, but specialized paper is also more expensive than 20-pound bond. Be aware that text printed on textured paper can be hard to read if the texture of the paper is too extreme. If you plan to photocopy your publication and want to use a paper size other than letter (8.5 by 11 inches) or legal (8.5 by 14 inches), make sure the photocopiers you have in mind for the job can handle that paper size.

Images

Images add to a publication's eye appeal and, in the case of maps and diagrams, can often convey an idea more efficiently than words. However, a typical design error is to use too many images. One photograph of a kindly librarian assisting a health consumer sends the message that your library is willing to help the public; three photographs of roughly the same scene sends the message that your publication is padded.

Decorative images (such as bullets, lines, borders, boxes, and shading) can enhance a publication by separating sections or emphasizing points. Nonetheless, beware of overkill. You don't want so many decorative boxes and lines that your publication ends up looking like a maze.

Clipart can enhance a publication, but be careful not to use inappropriate clipart. Party balloons or smiling clowns probably have no place on an AIDS brochure. Also watch out for overused clipart. How many times have you seen the Microsoft clipart image of the duck raring back to smash a computer with a hammer? How many times do you want to see it again? Good, fresh clipart can be found for free on the Internet, but make sure that any free clipart you download is actually free of copyright. Just because a Web site tells you its clipart images of Bugs Bunny are free of copyright does not mean that they are. Buying clipart from reliable sources on the Web, or buying clipart (on CD-ROM) from art shops or computer stores, may be the best way to get quality, copyright-free clipart that has not been used ad nauseam.

If your budget allows, commissioning original artwork from a professional graphic artist is a great way to go. Good graphic artists do not come cheap, so make sure you know what you are getting before you buy. Ask to see previous examples of a graphic artist's work, and get a firm estimate of what the finished artwork will cost. Be aware that changes to the finished art ("This is great, but can you put the tree on the left instead of the right?") will cost you.

Image quality is an important consideration. All images lose some quality in the process of being reproduced. A blurry photograph does not get better after a trip through the scanner or photocopier—it only gets worse. It is better not to use an image than to use a poor quality image, no matter how good the image *almost* is.

Consistency

When you plan to create more than one related publication, consistency in appearance can help convey the message that all these different publications are related in some way. You can achieve consistency by using the same color of paper for all your consumer health publications, or by using the same general format, layout, and typefaces. A shared front-page logo can also help to tie the publications together.

Desktop-Publishing Software

If you are creating a reasonably simple publication—perhaps a bibliography of health information resources printed on 8.5-by-11-inch paper—you may not need to use desktop-publishing software at all. Word-processing software, such as WordPerfect or Microsoft Word, may be quite up to the task, especially if you are using an up-to-date version of the software.

The next step up from word-processing software is Microsoft's Publisher. If you have Microsoft Office on your computer, you may already have Publisher; if not, Publisher can be purchased for well under $100. Besides being inexpensive, Publisher has the twin virtues of being easy to learn yet sophisticated enough to produce good looking publications that would be impossible to create with word-processing software. Publisher's wizards make it easy to create flyers, tri-fold brochures, and other publications, but the software also allows you to develop a publication from scratch or to change elements of a publication created from a wizard.

As useful as they may be, low-end desktop-publishing software packages cannot compete with professional-quality packages, such as Adobe PageMaker and QuarkXPress. These software packages can produce stunning results, but they are relatively costly and difficult to master. Taking a formal course of instruction in PageMaker or QuarkXPress is not a bad idea if you wish to use either software package to its full potential.

Printing

When it actually comes time to print a consumer health publication, one must usually choose between in-house and professional printing.

In-house printing using a photocopier or laser printer is often the least expensive way to produce a small run of a publication. It also has the advantage of allowing you to publish only the number of copies you need on a just-in-time basis. With the spread of color photocopiers and color printers, it is now possible to produce color publications in-house, though such publications will cost more than black-and-white publications. The disadvantages of in-house publications are that they may not look as nice as professionally printed publications, you are limited to certain paper sizes, and chores like folding, collating, and stapling all have to be done in-house.

Before running off large numbers of photocopies in-house, check the cost of having the copying done at a commercial photocopying shop such as Kinko's. For large runs, using a photocopying shop may be less expensive than in-house photocopying and, depending on the quality and robustness of your in-house copiers, result in better looking publications.

For large runs, sending publications to a professional printing shop can be less expensive than photocopying; plus, the finished publication usually looks better than one produced by photocopy machines. When you send a publication to a professional printing shop, the more copies you have printed at one time, the lower the cost per copy. Making a realistic estimate of how many copies you will actually use prevents either costly return trips to the printer or the need to send boxes of unused copies to the recycler. Few professional printing shops can produce documents on the spur of the moment, which means that you must plan ahead. You can greatly reduce the cost of professional printing by using desktop publishing programs (see above) to produce camera-ready copy.

If you are planning to work with a professional printer, it is crucial that you meet with the printer in advance. Even if you are using a noncommercial printing shop that is part of your home institution, keep in mind that you are negotiating a business deal and that you must know exactly what you will get and how much it will cost before any printing begins. Some questions to ask a printer include:

- What is the cost for black and white versus spot color versus four-color printing?
- What sizes, weights, and colors of paper are available and what do they cost?
- Are folding and stapling included in the cost?
- What is the set-up fee for the initial printing? Will this fee be waived if I come back for a second run of the same publication?
- What is the cost for 100, 500, 1,000, copies?
- What constitutes camera-ready copy?
- Do you accept publications on disk?
- If so, what desktop-publishing software packages are acceptable to you?
- When will the job be ready?
- Will you deliver the job or do I need to pick it up?
- Do you have any suggestions for making this publication look better or making it less costly to produce?

Don't hesitate to use a printer as a source of advice. A knowledgeable, experienced printer can come up with ideas that will save you money and result in better looking publications.

Distributing a Consumer Health Publication

Creating a consumer health publication is nothing more than an intellectual exercise if the publication never reaches those who need it. Effective distribution—in print and/or on the Web—requires at least as much thought and effort as writing the publication in the first place.

When it comes to distributing printed consumer health publications, the object is to put copies where the target audience will find them. In libraries, this strategy generally means displaying publications on some type of stand or rack near the library entrance or reference desk. Given the general interest in consumer health publications, however, there are many places besides the library where such publications will be used and appreciated. Possible places of distribution include:

- Hospitals, clinics, and doctors' offices
- Campus health centers and student union buildings.
- Social service agencies (public-assistance offices, homeless shelters)
- Retail businesses (grocery stores, shopping malls)
- Corporate settings (human-resources offices, corporate wellness centers)
- Churches

- Senior-citizen centers and retirement homes
- Elementary and secondary schools
- Community centers

The special nature of some consumer health publications may suggest a logical place of distribution. Obviously, Spanish-language consumer health publications might best reach their audience if they are displayed at such businesses as Hispanic grocery stores, *librerias*, and so on, while a publication on breast cancer might find an appreciative audience at a neighborhood beauty parlor.

At every site where you hope to display and distribute your publications, you will need to convince somebody to give you the required space. Space is a precious commodity, so you will not always succeed in placing your publications at every desired location. When you do get space, you may have to supply a rack or some other piece of display hardware. You will also need to establish an on-site contact who will call you whenever the supply of publications runs low. Even with such contacts, occasional tours of your distribution points will be necessary to ensure that your publications are in stock and on display.

Creating a consumer health publication from whole cloth is a lot of work, but it is a one-time job. Getting that publication to its audience requires an on-going commitment from everyone involved. Unless an organization is satisfied with using consumer health publications as nothing more than "See What a Good Thing We Did" trophies, administrators must be willing and able to commit resources to the long-term job of distributing those publications to those who need them.

Distribution Via the Web

The Web is a wonderful way to distribute consumer health publications:

- The cost of distribution is low.
- The audience is worldwide.
- Updating is easy.
- You never run out of copies.

On the other hand, there are some notable downsides to the Web:

- Web-based publications are useless to those who cannot or will not use the Web.
- The Web is so vast that making your intended audience aware of your publications is difficult.
- Organizing and maintaining a collection of Web-based publications requires considerable labor.

From Print to Web

One way to distribute consumer health publications via the Web is to take existing print publications and put them, as is, onto the Web, but there are drawbacks to this "shovelware" approach. First of all, the best Web publications are interactive, while print publications are static. This means that when a print publication migrates to the Web, it is best to include such enhancements as links to related resources (such as other informational Web sites or support-group homepages) and feedback features (such as mailto links and feedback forms).

Existing print publications can be scanned and put on the Web, but this approach doesn't always work as neatly as one might imagine:

- There is always some loss of visual quality when a publication is scanned.
- Scanning publications requires considerable labor. Not only does the scanning itself take time, but proofing scanned documents and tweaking them so they look presentable requires considerable effort and skill.
- Often, the dimensions of scanned publications do not translate well to the dimensions of computer monitors.
- Scanned publications do not have the interactive features of the best Web publications.

The alternative to scanning an existing print publication is to recreate it as a Web publication in HTML format. Converting a print publication into HTML is labor-intensive even if you can cut and paste the text from an electronic file. Because most desktop-publishing (and some word-processing) software packages allow you to save a document as HTML, you may be able to avoid much of the labor of converting a document. However, even with such "Save As HTML" features, you will still need to edit the HTML version of each document to get it just right.

Web to Print

If a consumer health publication was originally created for the Web, you do not face the problem of converting it from print form. However, many Web publications do not print well. The best solution to this problem is to have an on-screen version of the publication in HTML format and a printable version in some other format. By far, the most popular format for printing Web publications is Adobe's Portable Data Format (.pdf). The advantages of .pdf files are that they print out exactly as they were laid out and that Adobe Acrobat Reader (the software needed to view and print .pdf files) is freely and widely available via the Web. One downside of .pdf files is that those who do not have Adobe Acrobat Reader on their computers must download and install it in order to view .pdf publications—often a daunting task for those not overly comfortable with computers. Second, if you wish to save your publications as .pdf files, you will need to purchase the complete Adobe Acrobat software package, which currently retails for about $250 (somewhat less for academic institutions).

See the section "Draw Attention to your Web Site" in Chapter 10 for information on how to make the public aware of your Web-based publications.

10
Building Successful Consumer Health Web Sites for Your Users

A good Web site[1] is more like a garden than a sculpture. Like both a garden and a sculpture, a good Web site requires planning and a lot of initial work to bring the creation to life. Unlike a sculpture, however, a Web site does not have an ending point at which the work is unveiled and the creator goes on to the next project. Like a garden, a Web site needs continual tending if it is not to disintegrate into a ruin.

So one requirement for building a good consumer health Web site is a long-term commitment to the Sisyphean task of tending the site day in and day out: planting new growth, fixing up areas that fall into disrepair, and weeding that which is no longer vital. Of course before you can begin tending a Web site you must do the substantial work of designing the site so that your users can successfully navigate it. And you must stock the site with useful content that, ideally, has not been done to death by dozens of other sites. Even with all the above done and done well, getting people to visit your Web site remains a considerable task—just look at all the heavily advertised start-up Web sites that have failed because they could not get enough Web surfers to knock on their flashy front doors.

Despite all of the work involved, a Web site is still a great way to get information to healthcare consumers. The tricks to succeeding are to:

- Know your Web site's purpose.
- Understand your users.
- Provide quality content.
- Follow a few basic rules of good Web site design.

Know Your Purpose

Before engaging in the work of creating a consumer health Web site, you should have a clear purpose in mind. Too often, a Web site is launched with-

---

1. A Web site can consist of as little as a single Web page or run to thousands of pages. It may well be that your consumer health "Web site" will be a single page, or handful of pages, within your organization's larger Web site.

out a clear purpose or with a purpose determined either by fiat from above or by guesswork from the trenches. A much better way to determine a purpose for a consumer health Web site is to begin by seeking input from those the site is intended to serve. Asking questions, conducting surveys, observing what kinds of consumer health information your intended users seek and how they go about seeking it—these and other feedback-gathering techniques can help focus the purpose of a consumer health Web site before the first line of HTML is ever written. Used wisely, user feedback will go a long way toward making a consumer health Web site something that is used rather than useless. (See the next section, "Understand Your Users," for more on the important topic of user feedback.)

When you do settle on a purpose, make sure that it is not too ambitious. For example:

> The purpose of the Corday Public Library Consumer Health Web site is to serve as the Internet's leading one-stop shop for consumer health information.

That is a grand purpose, all right, but not one that you will come close to achieving without millions—lots and lots of millions—of dollars to spend on staff, hardware, software, and advertising. Excessively ambitious purposes produce Web sites that do a lot of things poorly and nothing well. Aim high, but be reasonable:

> The purpose of this Web site is to help patrons of the Corday Public Library locate consumer health resources in CPL and the local community.

This is a more modest purpose, but one that is doable. Besides, once you have achieved your modest goal you can always revise upward and build on your success.

Understand Your Users

When you create print publications you must consider your audience. The same is true when you design, or redesign, a consumer health Web site. While the potential users of any Web site are, in theory, everyone on the Internet, it is unlikely that the whole wired world will come calling at your Web site. Who, then, are your primary users? The people who walk through the doors of your library every day? The patients and families of your hospital or clinic? Healthcare providers looking for information to pass along to their patients? Is your typical user more likely to be a senior, a parent, or a school child, or do your users come equally from all age groups? Is English a foreign or second language to a significant number of your users? What health issues are of most concern to your users? Do your users tend to be experienced or inexperienced Web surfers? Will users most often access your Web site via slow dial-up Internet connections, or are they more likely to have high-speed access?

While it is impossible to know everything about everyone who uses your Web site, gathering feedback from even a small sampling of users—and responding intelligently to what this feedback tells you—allows you to create a more usable Web site than you could possibly create without feedback. And gathering feedback does not require a costly and time-consuming canvass of every potential user. In fact, noted Web-design expert Jakob Nielsen contends that conducting usability testing with more than five potential users is a waste of time and money.[2]

If you are planning to revise or expand an established Web site, one way to solicit user comments is via mailto links and feedback forms. Mailto links are so easy to create that you can (and should) put one on every page of your Web site. Feedback forms require more work to create, but they allow you to solicit more structured responses than you can get with mailto links.[3] Even so, good feedback forms should have at least one section where users are free to write whatever they wish. The one caveat about mailto links and feedback forms is that some person or persons on the staff must take on the responsibility of replying to users in a timely manner. Nothing says, "We don't care about you," quite so loudly as Web site administrators who never reply to user questions and comments. For mailto links and feedback forms to be effective, they must be easy for Web site visitors to find. Place such links in prominent locations on the homepage as well as on interior pages. Finally, there is nothing wrong with making mailto links and feedback forms a permanent feature of your Web site.

When undertaking a major redesign of an existing Web site, a good technique is to launch a beta-test Web site that runs parallel to the existing Web site. Links on the existing Web site invite users to try the beta Web site. Once at the beta Web site, visitors are given ample opportunity (via mailto links or feedback forms) to comment on what they like or do not like about the beta site. Because the beta site is in a test phase, it is possible to make changes based on visitor feedback without worrying that these changes will disorient regular users of the site. This technique also has the advantage of softening,

---

2. Nielsen, Jakob. "Why You Only Need to Test With 5 Users." *Alertbox*. March 19, 2000. *www.useit.com/alertbox/20000319.html*.

3. If you are interested in creating Web feedback forms, one easy solution is to use Zoomerang, a commercial Web service that allows you to quickly create feedback forms and easily track responses. Visit the Zoomerang Web site at *www.zoomerang.com* for more information. A similar form-support service is offered by Free & Clear at *www.freeandclear.nu*.

The Hathaway Medical Center Library Consumer Health Web Site

Included as part of this book are the various computer files comprising the consumer health Web site of the fictional Hathaway Medical Center Library. While not intended as an exact blueprint, this Web site suggests possible content and architecture for a consumer health Web site. Feel free to take from it that which suits you and ignore that which does not.

Some of the Web pages on the HMC Library Web site have real content and therefore look and function like genuine Web pages; other pages function more like placeholders and contain text describing content that could go on such a Web page. Our decisions on whether a Web page should be genuine or placeholder were based on which format best conveys the concept underlying that Web page.

With the exceptions of the "Search this Web site" box and the mailto links, everything on the HMC Library Web site is live—when you click on a link, something will happen.

---

for at least some users, the blow that always comes when a Web site undergoes a major redesign.

Another way to gather feedback is to hold formal usability-testing sessions with a few representative users. During such sessions you can ask participants about their likes, dislikes, wants, and so on. Even better, though, is to allow participants to navigate your Web site while you take notes on how they use the site and where they run into problems navigating it. While incentives such as free meals or small honoraria are often necessary to entice users to participate in formal usability-testing sessions, and while such sessions often require a one-to-one, or even two-to-one, staff-to-participant ratio, the insight you gain is well worth the time and cost. For an especially good article on the topic of gathering user feedback while redesigning a Web site, see "Usability Testing at the University of Arizona Library: How to Let the Users in on the Design."[4]

Provide Quality Content

Once you have decided on a purpose and considered your users, it is then possible to think about content. Other than content that simply mirrors that of another Web site, there are really only two kinds of content: original con-

---

4. Dickstein, Ruth, and Vicki Mills. "Usability Testing at the University of Arizona Library: How to Let the Users in on the Design." *Information Technology and Libraries* 19, no. 3 (September 2000):144–150. Also available online at *www.lita.org/ital/1903_mills.html*.

Disclaimers and Privacy Policies

If you have a Web site with any kind of health-related information on it, you should have a disclaimer. See Chapter 9 for advice on disclaimers.

Either as part of your disclaimer or as a separate Web page, you should have a privacy policy that tells users what you will and will not do with any information you might collect about them.

---

tent and links to other resources. The best Web sites do a good job of balancing both kinds of content.

Original Content

Original content is what too many Web sites lack—in large part because it is easier to make lots of links to lots of other sites than it is to come up with something useful and original to put on your own site. You should buck this trend and improve the quality of your Web site by including at least some appropriate original content.

One kind of original content you must provide is information about the Web site itself (such as purpose and policies) as well as about the site's developers, sponsors, and maintainers. (See "Use 'About'" in the section "Follow Basic Web Site Design Rules" later in this chapter.)

Converting your organization's existing consumer health publications from print to Web format is one way to beef up your Web site's original content. Along the same lines, you might seek permission from local hospitals, clinics, or health departments to convert their printed consumer health publications to Web format and mount the results on your Web site. Using existing print publications saves the work of writing new publications from scratch, but the process of converting a document from print to electronic format requires significant labor and expertise.

Repackaging information in a form that is more convenient, understandable, or accessible also falls under the heading of original content. Say, for example, that basic information about the seven hospitals serving your county is scattered across seven different institutional Web sites. You can create useful original content by pulling all this information together so that users can easily find and compare information about all seven hospitals on a single, well-organized Web page. For another example, you could take important health information that is written in highly technical language and translate it into language a lay reader can understand. Just be sure you put the repackaged information in your own words and cite the original source or sources as necessary.

Local Angle

The old axiom "local information is the hardest information to find" certainly holds true for consumer health information. One of the best ways to make a consumer health Web site truly useful and, at the same time, distinguish it from hundreds of similar sites is to emphasize the local angle. Depending on your Web site's purpose and primary users, local could be as small as a city neighborhood or larger than an entire state. The exact definition of *local* is not as important as the fact that you are providing your users with personally useful and important information that is not readily provided by countless other Web sites.

For example, you *could* list the "Seven Warning Signs of Cancer" on your Web site or, even more easily, make a link from your Web site to any of the many cancer-related Web sites that list the warning signs; however, this widely available information can be found by typing "seven warning signs of cancer" into just about any Web search engine. Of more use to your users would be a listing (with contact information) of hard-to-find local resources for cancer information, treatment, and support.

To determine what kind of local information is most needed, it helps to get feedback from your users. It is also worthwhile to scout other Web sites that originate in your local area to see what local consumer health information is or is not available. For example, a well-organized list of local hospitals and nursing homes (with addresses, phone numbers, and links to Web pages) could be a valuable addition to your consumer health Web site, but if a perfectly good list already exists on another local Web site, a link to the existing resource makes more sense than duplicating the other site's content.

In many cases, gathering local consumer health information means going beyond the Web. Because local health-related services and organizations may lack the resources or expertise needed to produce and maintain a Web presence, you will have to open up the phone book, scour the newspapers, and talk to local people to identify those health resources in your area that should be included in your consumer health Web site. If you are diligent in your efforts, your Web site can become, in effect, the surrogate Web presence for those local health resources that cannot mount their own Web sites.

Another aspect of the local approach is to focus not only on local health resources but on local health concerns as well. For example, if your local area is heavily industrialized, you might want to focus on health problems associated with pollution. Or if mosquito-borne disease is a serious problem in your area, then a focus on that topic would be appropriate. When you focus on local health issues, you may wish to feature both local and national (or even international) resources on those issues. After all, while featuring local resources is a good thing, this does not mean that you cannot also employ outside resources.

But what if there are too many local health concerns to cover them all? Then focus on as many of the most important ones as you can. Even focusing on one local health concern and doing a good job is better than covering a lot of health concerns poorly. It is better to be the site known for all the great content and links about Valley Fever than to be another anonymous Web site with dozens of the same predictable links to widely known health information resources that already appear on several thousand other Web sites.

A Web-based guide to the print and/or electronic consumer health resources available in or from your library or other institution is yet another type of original content to include on your Web site. Such a guide can be as simple as a brief list of important consumer health books in your collection, or it can be a major production that includes annotations, information about consumer health on the Web, and tips on evaluating consumer health information. Users often print guides of this type, so offering them in both HTML format for reading and .pdf format for printing is helpful.

Finally, you can always add original content by creating Web-based consumer health publications from scratch. Again, Chapter 9 provides tips for producing this type of content.

Links

Hyperlinks that move visitors from one Web page to another with a single click are one of the most powerful features of the Web. However, as the ten-year anniversary of the Web approaches, Web sites that are nothing more than repositories of links are old news. If you have some notion of creating a consumer health Web site that is distinguished by the sheer number of links it provides, that notion should vanish after you take a look at a few of the many biomedical megasites already filling that niche. (See the Megasite Project at *www.lib.umich.edu/megasite/toc.html* for information about health information megasites.) Not only is compiling large numbers of consumer health links futile because it is redundant, the amount of work involved in compiling, organizing, and maintaining so many links is staggering. If you want your users to have access to a broad range of health information, the best strategy is to make links to a few carefully chosen, consumer-oriented biomedical megasites that specialize in quantity *and* quality.

As for the links you choose to include on your Web site, go for quality. One way to achieve quality is to create links that point to information on local health resources and concerns. (See the "Local Angle" sidebar in this chapter.) Annotating the links you make to other Web sites is one of the best services you can provide for your users; rating the Web sites you link to can be similarly helpful, though chances are you will give most of them good ratings because you will not want to waste anyone's time by linking to inferior Web sites. Focusing your links on a few important health issues, rather than trying to cover everything, is another way to maintain quality.

Whatever number of links you choose to include on your site, every link needs to be checked regularly to make sure a linked site has not moved or folded. The best way to do this is to use link-checking software that tests every link on your Web site and reports any problems. Advanced Web site authoring software packages (such as DreamWeaver and FrontPage) include link checkers. It is also possible to acquire stand-alone link-checking software programs. One of the more popular of these is Xenu's *Link Sleuth*, which can be downloaded for free from *www.home.snafu.de/tilman/xenulink.html*.

Follow Basic Web Site Design Rules

There is no such thing as a perfect Web site that everyone finds equally appealing and equally easy to navigate. Web site design is such a highly subjective art that sites appearing on one Web-design expert's list of award-winning sites can end up on another expert's "Worst of the Web" list. Even if you cannot achieve perfection and please everyone, you can make your Web site more usable by adhering to a few basic design principles.

Remember that Simple Is Better

Flashy, eye-catching Web sites make people say "Wow." For about ten seconds. Then these sites often prove to be nothing more than pretty frustrations. The simpler the design, the more likely users will find what they are looking for. Avoid gimmicks, such as gratuitous frames, huge graphics, blinking text, bandwidth-clogging scripts, and meaningless animations. A well-done, simple site will serve you better than a would-be flashy site that, at the end of the day, will never flash as brightly as the multimillion-dollar, bleeding-edge commercial sites that vie to impress jaded Web users.

Figure 10.1 shows the homepage for the Argus Clearinghouse (*www. clearinghouse.net*), which is one of the most highly regarded directories on the Web. Every page on this site is a testament to the effectiveness of simple, clean design.

Figure 10.1: Argus Clearinghouse Homepage

The Internet's Premier Research Library
A Selective Collection of Topical Guides

The **Argus**Clearinghouse

Navigation

Search/Browse

Internet Searching
Center

Site Information

FAQ

Submit a Guide

Digital Librarian's
Award

Ratings System

Contact Us

Categories

Arts & Humanities

Business & Employment

Communication

Computers & Information
Technology

Education

Engineering

Environment

Government & Law

Health & Medicine

Places & Peoples

Recreation

Science & Mathematics

Social Sciences & Social
Issues

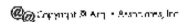 Copyright © Argus Associates, Inc.

Follow Web Conventions

Though the Web has been in existence less than ten years, some Web conventions are already firmly established. Like many conventions and standards that we follow (such as the "qwerty" keyboard), Web conventions are not always the most efficient way of doing things; nonetheless, adherence to Web conventions will make a site easier to navigate—at least for those users who have some familiarity with the Web. As a general rule, if you perceive that most of the big-name Web sites you visit (for example, Amazon.com, Yahoo!, eBay, CNN.com, and New York Public Library) adhere to a particular Web-design convention, then you should follow their lead unless you have an extremely good reason not to.

Create Multiple Access Points

The great thing about a Web site is that you can easily create multiple access points to a single thing, making it possible for users to find what they want even if they do not follow the route you might anticipate. Typical Web site access points include subject classification, a site map, an alphabetical list of resources, and a site-specific search engine.

SUBJECT CLASSIFICATION

The trick to using subject classification on a Web site is to choose subject headings that users understand. On a consumer health Web site, using "**Cancer**" as a subject heading makes more sense than using "**Oncology**." Even more sensible is to use both "**Cancer**" and "**Oncology**" as subject headings and have both headings point users to the same resources. Similarly, listing a single resource under multiple subject headings is often appropriate. A link to your "**Local Cancer Resources**" Web page might, for instance, be found under the categories of "**Wellness**" *and* "**Diseases & Conditions**" *and* "**Local Resources**."

SITE MAP

A site map lays out the architecture of a Web site so that users can see at a glance how the site is organized. Site maps can be extremely effective tools for helping users find their way, which is why most large Web sites have them. One caveat: users sometimes click on "Site Map" hoping to find an actual map to, or floor plan of, a physical location. For this reason it is considerate to include links on your site map to direct users to actual maps to, and floor plans of, your facility.

Figure 10.2, an example from the National Center for Biotechnology Information (*www.ncbi.nlm.nih.gov/Sitemap*), combines a site map (left-hand column) and an alphabetical list (gray background) on a single page.

Figure 10.2: National Center for Biotechnology Information Site Map

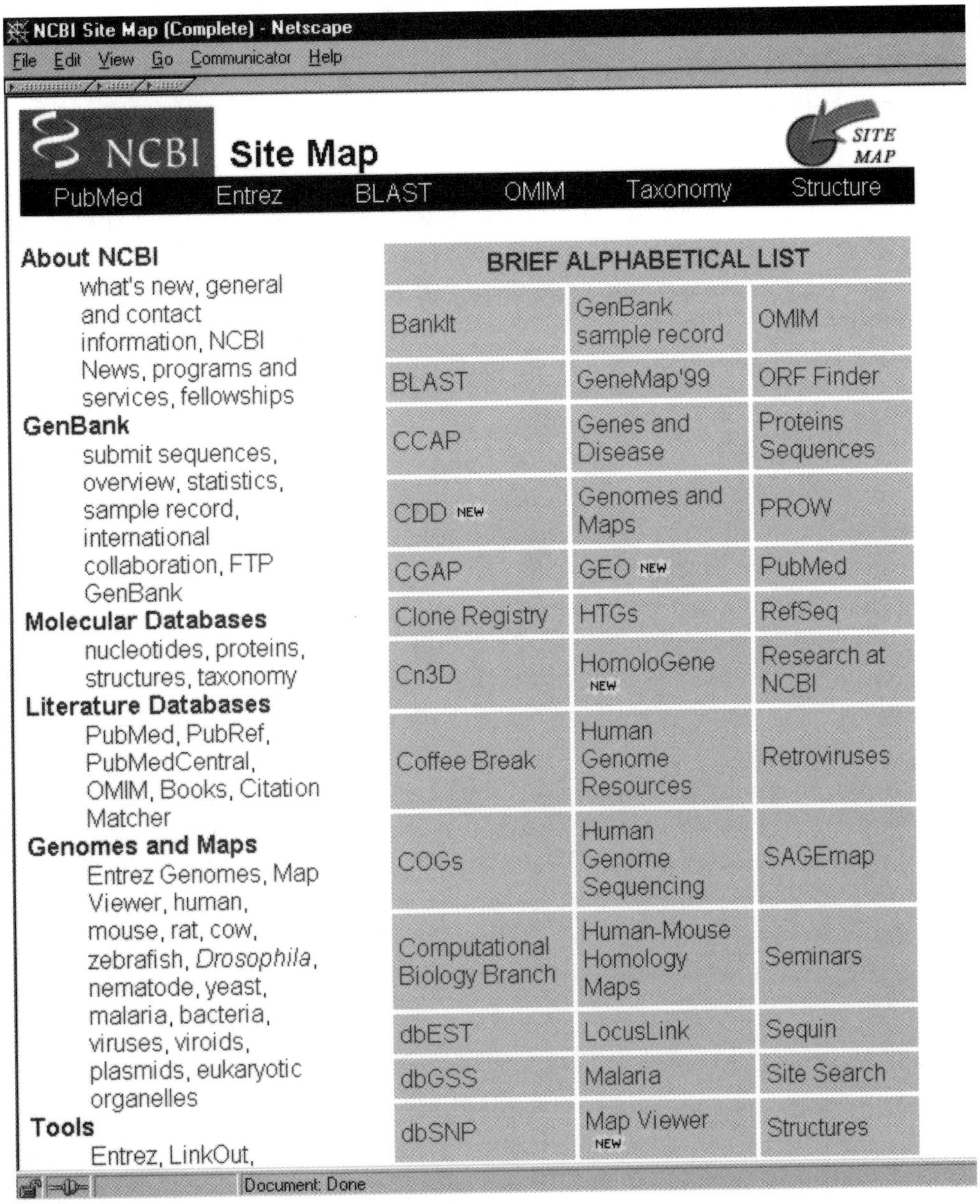

NCBI Site Map (Complete) - Netscape

File Edit View Go Communicator Help

NCBI Site Map

SITE MAP

PubMed   Entrez   BLAST   OMIM   Taxonomy   Structure

About NCBI

what's new, general and contact information, NCBI News, programs and services, fellowships

GenBank

submit sequences, overview, statistics, sample record, international collaboration, FTP GenBank

Molecular Databases

nucleotides, proteins, structures, taxonomy

Literature Databases

PubMed, PubRef, PubMedCentral, OMIM, Books, Citation Matcher

Genomes and Maps

Entrez Genomes, Map Viewer, human, mouse, rat, cow, zebrafish, *Drosophila*, nematode, yeast, malaria, bacteria, viruses, viroids, plasmids, eukaryotic organelles

Tools

Entrez, LinkOut,

BRIEF ALPHABETICAL LIST		
BankIt	GenBank sample record	OMIM
BLAST	GeneMap'99	ORF Finder
CCAP	Genes and Disease	Proteins Sequences
CDD NEW	Genomes and Maps	PROW
CGAP	GEO NEW	PubMed
Clone Registry	HTGs	RefSeq
Cn3D	HomoloGene NEW	Research at NCBI
Coffee Break	Human Genome Resources	Retroviruses
COGs	Human Genome Sequencing	SAGEmap
Computational Biology Branch	Human-Mouse Homology Maps	Seminars
dbEST	LocusLink	Sequin
dbGSS	Malaria	Site Search
dbSNP	Map Viewer NEW	Structures

Document: Done

Alphabetical List of Resources

An alphabetical list of resources on a Web site works exactly like a traditional book index and is a real help to those who are more comfortable navigating a book than a Web site. As with a book index, the key is to provide adequate cross-references so that users can find what they are looking for regardless of what terminology they use (in other words, *cancer*, *neoplasm*, *tumor*, *oncology* should all lead users to the same set of cancer-related resources).

Site-Specific Search Engine

A site-specific search engine allows users to search a single Web site by keyword. Be sure to label a site-specific search engine so that users know it searches only the site they are currently visiting, not the entire Internet. For any Web site of more than 50 pages, a site-specific search engine is a necessity, not an option.

Follow Conventions for Navigation Tools

Navigation tools (aka "nav bars") are icons or text that link visitors to important pages or features of a Web site. By convention, navigation tools go on the left-hand side of a page, across the top of a page, or in both locations. The look of navigation tools usually remains constant from one Web page to the next, though it is good practice to "gray out" or remove the navigation tool representing the page being displayed (for example on the page "Diseases and Conditions," gray out or remove the navigation icon that links to "Diseases and Conditions").

As shown in Figure 10.3, the National Center for Biotechnology Information (*www.ncbi.nlm.nih.gov*) follows the convention of placing navigation tools on the left and top of each Web page. This is an example of a convention that is so entrenched that Web designers break it at their own risk. Note that it is typical to place image-based navigation tools across the top of the page and text-format tools down the left-hand side.

Consider Other Page Layout Conventions

Navigation tools usually go at the top of a Web page because they are important. Important things go at the top of a page because users can see them without scrolling down. Filling the tops of Web pages with huge graphics, Web site counters, meaningless Web awards, or colossal-sized text is a bad use of prime real estate. However, a concise, descriptive page title should appear near the top of every Web page.

The bottom of a Web page is the standard location for mailto links of the "Contact Us" variety (though there is nothing wrong with placing additional mailto links in other locations on a page as well). If a Web page includes such

Figure 10.3: National Center for Biotechnology Information Homepage

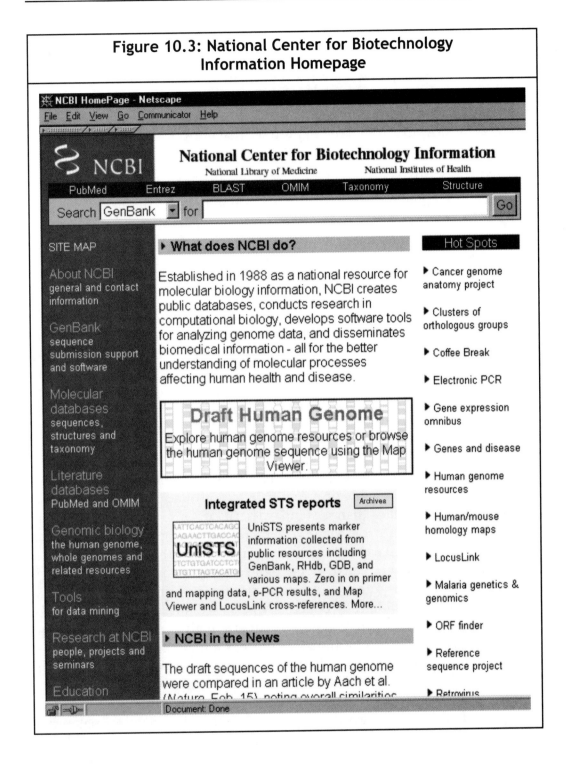

information as a physical address, phone numbers, or information on when the page was last updated, this also typically goes at the bottom of the page.

In general, anything placed on the right-hand side of a Web page is in such danger of being cropped off by a small-sized monitor that nothing critically important goes on the right-hand side of a page. Even worse, many Web users do not know how to scroll to the right to see that cut-off part of the Web page.

Maintain a Consistent Style

As a rule, maintain a consistent style from one page to the next. If colors, images, themes, location of navigation tools, and general page layout remain consistent, it cues users to the fact that they have not clicked off your Web site and moved on to new cyber turf. Consistency also means that once users have figured out how to navigate one page on a site, they have figured it out for every page on that site.

Major sections of a Web site may break the consistency rule if there is a good reason to do so. For example, a "For Kids" section on a consumer health Web site might have a different, more age-appropriate, look from the rest of the site. Even when you choose to give some part or parts of your Web site a distinctive look, carrying over some variation of the colors, themes, images, and layout from the main Web site helps to tie the entire Web site together.

Ensure Readability of Text

The most important thing about text is that it should stand out from its background. Black text on a white or a very pale background is the best option. If you use something other than a standard serif or sans-serif font, the result may look very different from what you intended to those who lack that font on their computers. Relative size of text is important in that headings or titles should be larger than body text, but actual size is less important since that is largely at the mercy of screen and browser settings. Even so, do not use extremely small text. Boldface is effective when used sparingly. Italics can be hard to read on some monitors, so use that sparingly too. Do not underline plain text, as underlining traditionally indicates a hyperlink.

Though it has long been possible to make text links appear any color, in the early days of the Web unvisited text links were always blue and visited text links were always purple. While making text links some color other than blue is acceptable if there is a good reason for it, it is a bad idea to make non-linking text blue or purple. Users are so accustomed to links being blue or purple that they will automatically click on any text of these colors and become confused, impatient, or angry if their clicking leads them nowhere.

Use "About"

In part because of the influence of commercial Web sites, "**About**" has become the standard label for information about the creators of the Web site, the purpose of the Web site, Web site policies, contact information, staff directories, and disclaimers. Putting this type of information anywhere other than under "**About**" is certain to make that information harder for most visitors to find.

Provide a FAQ Page

FAQ (Frequently Asked Questions) is what many Web site visitors look for first when they need in-depth information. If visitors to your Web site frequently become confused over which resources have restricted access and which can be accessed by anyone, you would do well to provide this information as a question and answer within a FAQ. Or you might create a FAQ question and answer that covers the topic of who can get a library card, or how to order copies of documents. In every FAQ you should include a link where visitors can submit questions not answered in the FAQ.

Think About Your Users' Technology

Few who visit your Web site will have access to the latest and greatest technology, so you need to take this into consideration when designing your site.

One of the most important things to know about Web design is that one Web page will not look the same on every computer. The Web page that looks good enough to eat when viewed with the latest version of Internet Explorer on your 19-inch SVGA monitor may look like day-old scrambled eggs when seen through the haze of an old version of Netscape on a 13-inch monitor. To avoid creating a page that looks good on less than one percent of the computers using the Web, take a look at your Web page on a variety of computers and monitors. Also look at your page on as many different releases of Netscape and Internet Explorer as you can get your hands on. You may need to make adjustments to get your Web pages looking good on most computers and browsers.

Keep in mind that many Web users connect via slow telephone modems and use slow computers. If your pages take too long to download, users will quickly give up trying to access your site. This means that you must avoid loading up your Web site with huge images, sound files, and other Web bric-a-brac that makes pages load slowly. Such Web-design software as FrontPage and DreamWeaver provide estimates for how long a page will take to download at various connection speeds (such as 28.8K and 56K). A page should not take more than seven seconds to download at the connection speed available to the majority of your users.

Learning More About Web Site Design

It is impossible in the confines of this book to give more than a quick over-view of Web design. Because there are so many opinions on what constitutes good Web site design, and because there are thousands of self-styled Web gurus dispensing all manner of advice, it is also impossible to point to any one source and say, "This is the Bible of Web design." Even so, there are some guides to Web design that stand out.

If anyone is a true guru of good Web site design, it is Jakob Nielsen. Nielsen's 1996 "Top Ten Mistakes of Web Design" (*www.useit.com/alertbox/ 9605.html*), along with his more recent updates on this topic, has become something of a Ten-Commandments-in-Progress for Web site design. Nielsen's biweekly *Alertbox* columns (*www.useit.com/alertbox*) are essential read-ing, and his recent book *Designing Web Usability*[5] would be many a Web designer's answer to the question, "If you could have just one book on Web design."

For making a pretty good Web site great though, there is nothing as user-friendly as *Creating a Power Web Site: HTML, Tables, Imagemaps, Frames, and Forms* by Gail Junion-Metz and Brad Stephens, and published by our very own Neal-Schuman. This book comes with a Web-enabled CD-ROM and is a step-by-step guide to quickly and powerfully enhancing and upgrading your site.

Another invaluable help from the Neal-Schuman catalog is *Creating a Virtual Library: A How-To-Do-It Manual* by Frederick Stielow. Everything you need to know to transform the library for cyberspace from the ground up is here.

Jennifer Fleming's *Web Navigation: Designing the User Experience* pro-vides many real-world examples as it approaches the topic of Web design from a user-centric point of view.[6]

A very friendly and thorough book on Web design is *The Non-Designer's Web Book*.[7] Its coverage of Web images is especially useful.

The Web4Lib discussion group (moderated by Roy Tennant) is a reliable source of information on both Web design and the more technical aspects of

---

5. Nielsen, Jakob. *Designing Web Usability: The Practice of Simplicity*. Indianapolis: New Riders, 2000.

6. Fleming, Jennifer. *Web Navigation: Designing the User Experience*. Sebastopol, Calif.: O'Reilly, 1998.

7. Williams, Robin, and John Tollett. *The Non-Designer's Web Book: An Easy Guide to Creating, Designing, and Posting Your Own Web Site*. 2d ed. Berkeley, Calif.: Peachpit Press, 2000.

maintaining Web sites. The Web4Lib homepage is *http://sunsite.berkeley/eduWeb4Lib*.

"Web Design for Librarians" (*http://scc01.rutgers.edu/SCCHome/policies/web.htm*) provides annotated links to several dozen Web sites that address issues of interest to librarian Web designers.

A related issue is the accessibility of your Web site to disabled users. The leading tool on the Web for evaluating the accessibility of Web pages is the Center for Applied Special Technology's Bobby (*www.cast.org/bobby*). A free service, Bobby produces a detailed report of all accessibility problems on any Web page that you ask it to examine. The downloadable version of Bobby will produce a report on an entire Web site.

Draw Attention to Your Web Site

In the big ocean of the Web, it is easy for a little boat of a consumer health Web site to go unnoticed. Here are some practical steps you can take to catch the attention of the Web-surfing public:

Provide a link from an institutional homepage: Chances are your consumer health Web site is a spin-off from, or a division of, a larger institutional Web site. If so, it is ideal to have a prominent link pointing directly from the institutional homepage to your consumer health Web site; if you cannot get a link from the homepage, try for links from as many interior pages as you can wrangle.

Produce handouts and make them readily available: Print-based publications are good for making walk-in clientele aware of your Web presence. Besides the usual signs, flyers, and brochures, consider printing up business cards or Rolodex cards that provide the name of the site, a description (perhaps brief) of the site's purpose, and the site's URL. These cards can be handed out at classes and meetings or offered to the public from card holders placed on public service desks. Finally, whatever print formats you use to spread the word about your consumer health Web site, this word will spread further if you can get your printed promotional material distributed or displayed in clinics, community centers, and other likely spots frequented by potential users of your Web site.

Get your Web site mentioned in appropriate print and broadcast media: This is another good way to make potential users aware of the resource. Newsletters and special-focus newspapers (such as neighborhood or ethnic newspapers) are easier to crack than big commercial newspapers, radio, and television. A large part of the problem with commercial print and broadcast media outlets is that most have their own Web sites and so, in their eyes, carrying news about your consumer health Web site is providing aid and comfort to the competition. Of course if news outlets will not spread the news of your Web site for free, they are always willing to sell you advertisements—an effective strategy if your budget allows.

Promote your consumer health Web site on appropriate listservs, newsgroups, and online support groups: If possible, promote your Web site to professionals (for example, healthcare providers and librarians) as well as to healthcare consumers.

Notify major Internet search engines and directories of the existence of your consumer health Web site: For example, **Yahoo!** (*www.yahoo.com*) has a link called "How to Suggest A Site" and **Lycos** (*www.lycos.com*) has a link called "Add Your Site to Lycos." While links like these make it easy to send information about your Web site to Internet search engines and directories, there is no guarantee that your Web site will be listed. Also, be aware that most for-profit Internet search engines and directories give preference to Web sites that pay to be listed. Even if your site gets listed, it will not be featured as prominently as, for example, the heavily advertised **drmoneybags.com** site. There are hundreds of for-profit companies in the business of marketing Web sites. A few of these companies are legitimate; most take your money and do little or nothing. Do your homework before giving anyone money to market your Web site, and beware of any company that *guarantees* it can get your Web site listed on **Yahoo!**, **Lycos**, and similar sites.

Consider using metadata: The use of metadata *may* increase the chances that users will find the consumer health resources you put on the Web, though there is evidence that major Internet search engines ignore metadata altogether. On the other hand, metadata are valuable for cataloging and other purposes. If you are interested in using metadata on your Web site, a good starting place is the **Dublin Core Metadata Initiative** at *www.purl.org/dc*.

Announce your consumer health Web site to other Web sites that are likely to make links to it. Potential Web sites to contact include those belonging to health-related associations and societies, government agencies, hospitals, libraries, schools, support groups, and for-profit businesses. Be sure to contact sites in your local area. In return for a link to your site, you may be asked to make a link back to the other site.

Index

About the Authors

Since December 1997 **Donald A. Barclay**, MA, MLIS, has been the Assistant Director for the Health Informatics Education Center at the Houston Academy of Medicine–Texas Medical Center Library. Prior to that, he held positions at the University of Houston and New Mexico State University. Educated at Boise State University and the University of California at Berkeley, he has published books and journal articles both on library topics as well as on the literature of the American West. He lives on Galveston Island, Texas, with his wife, Darcie R. Barclay, and their daughter, Mary Elizabeth.

Deborah D. Halsted, MLS, MA, is the Director of Library Operations at the Houston Academy of Medicine–Texas Medical Center Library. While at the library, she has managed numerous consumer health information projects, including the Jesse H. Jones Community Information Service, the CHIA (Consumer Health Information for Asians) project, and several consumer and public health projects sponsored by the National Library of Medicine. She has also served the library as the Outreach Coordinator for the National Network of Libraries of Medicine, South Central Region. Halsted is an active member of the Medical Library Association, the South Central Chapter of the Medical Library Association, and the TeXPEC (Texas Partnership for End of Life Care) Gulf Coast.

	DATE DUE		